ST PA - 44.

wr

Borr

Dama

Borrow

Fines ch.

CAN YOU AVOID CANCER?

CAN YOU AVOID cancer ?

An investigation by Peter Goodwin

BRITISH BROADCASTING CORPORATION

Peter Goodwin is a freelance science
broadcaster working with the BBC
External Services. He is also producer
of *Auditorium*, the cassette audio
medical updating service for hospital
doctors, and UK correspondent to the
Physicians Radio Network of America.

His previous books are *Future World*
(1979) and *Nuclear War: The Facts* (1981).
He has acted as consultant on two
BBC Television productions:
A Guide to Armageddon (1982)
and *Threads* (1984).

Peter Goodwin lives in London with his
actress wife and four daughters.

The BBC Continuing Education Television series,
Can You Avoid Cancer?, produced by Anna Jackson,
was first broadcast on BBC1 from June 1984

First published 1984
Published by the British Broadcasting Corporation
35 Marylebone High Street, London W1M 4AA

This book is set in 10/12 Plantin Linotron 202
by Phoenix Photosetting, Chatham
Printed in England by Mackays of Chatham Ltd

ISBN 0 563 21062 1

Contents

Introduction

If present trends continue one in five of us will die from cancer, the biggest killer disease (after heart disease) in the Western world. Must we simply accept this frightening prospect or can we do anything about it? Certainly research has not yet resulted in any breakthroughs which suggest that a radical new cure is just around the corner. In fact there is very little hope of any major discoveries during the foreseeable future which will revolutionise treatment, even though there may be some dramatic individual success stories.

But a mass of scientific evidence is emerging which seems to prove that cancer is by no means inevitable and that every one of us has the opportunity of making changes in our life-style and diet which offer good hope of greatly reducing our chances of getting this disease. In the following pages I shall explain why many scientists are now convinced that a small number of simple, practical steps should be urged on people in order to help them avoid cancer. We do not yet have all the answers and it may be many years before all the i's are dotted and the t's crossed. But by considering the scientific evidence, and the scientific doubts, that have been gathered so far, you will at least be able to judge for yourself.

Acknowledgments

The idea of writing this book arose from radio interviews I recorded with Professor Sir Richard Doll and Mr Richard Peto after publication of their 1981 report to the American Office of Technology Assessment on *The Causes of Cancer*. I owe a debt of gratitude to these Oxford scientists, as I do to Surgeon Captain T. L. Cleave of the Royal Navy whom I interviewed in 1977 and who planted the seed of understanding in my mind that many of our 'Western diseases' could be prevented. Invaluable discussions with Dr Andy Haines of the Northwick Park Hospital, London and at the newly formed European Organisation for Cancer Prevention in Brussels made the idea gel and my introduction to BBC producer Anna Jackson made it possible to publish the book in conjunction with a major television series, for which I am also thankful.

Dr Leo Kinlen of Oxford exhaustively refereed my original manuscript and provided many essential leads and scientific facts. In the later stages, Dr Kinlen and Sir Richard Doll contributed yet more painstaking work advising on factual accuracy, and although they are not responsible for any errors of fact or balance that may remain, their assistance has been invaluable. My thanks are also due to Dr A. B. Miller of the University of Toronto, Canada; Mr Denis Burkitt of Stroud, Gloucestershire; Dr Michael Waterfield and Dr Teich of the Imperial Cancer Research Fund in London; David Gee, National Health and Safety Officer, G.M.B.A.T.U.; and Dr Sheila Bingham of the Dunn Clinical Nutrition Centre, Cambridge, all of whom contributed ideas, comments and information, and to the many other scientists who have helped me prepare this investigation.

The book was only possible because of the co-operation, love, and moral support of my wife, Cleo, and children Paula, Cleotilda, Karen Louise, and Sarah Jane.

Last, but by no means least, I wish to thank my editor at BBC Publications, Jennie Allen, whose effort and input to the project were tremendous.

Peter Goodwin 1984

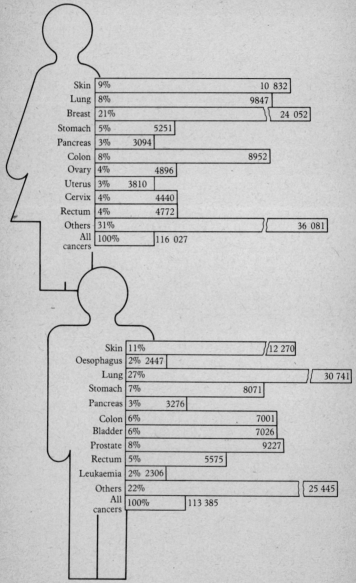

Skin	9%	10 832
Lung	8%	9847
Breast	21%	24 052
Stomach	5%	5251
Pancreas	3%	3094
Colon	8%	8952
Ovary	4%	4896
Uterus	3%	3810
Cervix	4%	4440
Rectum	4%	4772
Others	31%	36 081
All cancers	100%	116 027

Skin	11%	12 270
Oesophagus	2%	2447
Lung	27%	30 741
Stomach	7%	8071
Pancreas	3%	3276
Colon	6%	7001
Bladder	6%	7026
Prostate	8%	9227
Rectum	5%	5575
Leukaemia	2%	2306
Others	22%	25 445
All cancers	100%	113 385

Fig 1 Incidence of the 10 most common types of cancer in the UK in 1980.
(Figures supplied by the Cancer Research Campaign.)

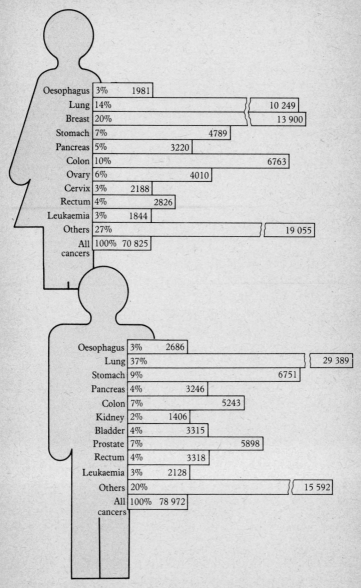

Fig 2 The 10 most common causes of cancer death in the UK in 1982.
(Figures supplied by the Cancer Research Campaign.)

1 Why cancer is not inevitable

It is important to realise that a wonder cure for cancer is not just around the corner. The battle doctors are waging to try to improve cure rates is a long, slow struggle – with no improvement at all, according to a recent British review, in the commonest of all Western cancers, lung cancer, since the 1950s. Great Britain leads the world in certain aspects of the 'cancer deaths league table'. Thirty eight per cent of all cancer deaths among men in Britain are from lung cancer – more than in America, or any other country. Hardly any of these deaths would occur if we did not smoke cigarettes, and it is perhaps appropriate that some of the most comprehensive scientific work which established the link between smoking and lung cancer was carried out in Britain.

Since the 1950s, medical scientists looking for other causes of cancer have found that some of the most important clues come from comparisons between one country and another, particularly between the affluent West, as typified by, say, the United States, and the developing world, where regions such as Africa have proved to be the fountain of many new ideas about the causes of cancer and other diseases. A black American man living in the city of Detroit, for example, is about 10 times more likely to die from cancer of the colon (the large bowel) than a black Nigerian man living in Ibadan. He is seven times more likely to die from cancer of the rectum than his African brother in Ibadan, a staggering 50 times more likely to experience premature death from lung cancer, and he faces a four-fold greater risk of dying from cancer of the pancreas or the larynx. These men share a similar racial, and therefore genetic, background, yet their cancer risks are completely different. In fact, all the cancers which are common in America, Britain and many West European countries are rare in less developed countries such as Nigeria. On the other

Table I Comparison of cancer rates for Africans in Ibadan, Nigeria, and for both blacks and whites in Detroit, USA. (Figures are for men unless otherwise stated.)

| Primary site of cancer | Annual incidence per million people below 65 years of age | | |
	Ibadan 1960–69 Africans	Detroit 1969–71 Blacks	Whites
Colon	34	353	33
Rectum	34	248	232
Liver	272	86	32
Pancreas	55	250	122
Larynx	37	149	141
Lung	27	1517	979
Prostate	134	577	232
Breast (women)	337	1105	1472
Cervix (women)	559	631	302
Womb (women)	42	208	441

(Adapted from *The Causes of Cancer* (OUP, 1981) by Doll and Peto.)

Table II High and low incidence areas for certain cancers. (Figures are for men unless otherwise stated.)

Site or origin of cancer	High incidence area	Low incidence area
Skin– chiefly non-melanoma	Queensland, Australia	Bombay, India
Gullet	Northeast Iran	Nigeria
Lung and bronchus	England	Nigeria
Stomach	Japan	Uganda
Cervix (women)	Colombia	Israel (Jewish)
Liver	Mozambique	England
Breast (women)	British Columbia, Canada	Israel (non-Jewish)
Colon	Connecticut, USA	Nigeria
Womb (women)	California, USA	Japan
Penis	Parts of Uganda	Israel (Jewish)

(Adapted from *The Causes of Cancer* (OUP, 1981) by Doll and Peto.)

hand, liver cancer, which is quite rare in Britain and America, is the commonest cancer among Nigerian men.

Among women of similar ethnic origins, the differences between Detroit and Ibadan are equally striking in terms of cancer incidence. Afro-American Detroit women are three times more likely to contract breast cancer and five times more likely to suffer from cancer of the body of the womb than the women of Ibadan, yet both cities report almost identical rates of cervical cancer. And even amongst young children the cancer rates vary, those in Ibadan suffering from a group of cancers called lymphosarcomas which are 30 times more common there than in Detroit.

The fact of the matter is that every cancer which is common in one place is found to be rare somewhere else. There are high and low incidence areas of every type of the disease, and although these often correspond to different countries, they can also be strikingly clear between different parts of the same country and between different groups of people in the same city. Asbestos workers, for example, suffer a markedly higher incidence of cancer of the lining of the lung (mesothelioma) than other people living in the same area who do not work in this industry. In this case a clear relationship has been firmly identified between the presence of asbestos fibres in inhaled air and the incidence of mesothelioma. Also, smokers who work with asbestos are much more likely to get lung cancer than smokers in other occupations. The *precise* degree to which asbestos is responsible for cancer deaths within the asbestos industry world-wide is subject to controversy, but it is clear that many cases of cancer would be prevented by removing humans totally from asbestos dust exposure. Whether this is a practical preventative measure to take or not is, of course, a matter for managements, unions and health officials, but the fact remains that asbestos dust is a specific cause of cancer which has been identified.

In the same way, the enormous differences in cancer incidence between Ibadan in Nigeria, and Detroit in the USA, can be explained in terms of the absence or presence of certain factors in these two cities. It almost goes without saying, for example, that the hugely greater incidence of lung cancer in Detroit is caused by the fact that cigarette smoking is a very common habit in the USA, but has only been adopted recently, and only then by a minority of citizens, in Ibadan. It takes 20 or 30 years for cigarette smoking to cause lung cancer, so countries like Nigeria will appear to be relatively immune from lung cancer for the time being, but can expect to see a future epidemic of this disease.

These general principles apply to comparisons between almost any two countries you care to mention. American women in the state of Iowa, USA, for example, have the lowest incidence of stomach cancer in the world; among Japanese men, to take an opposite extreme, the disease is 83 times more common. The city of Liverpool in the UK has the distinction of conferring the lowest risk in the world of a form of skin cancer known as melanoma on its inhabitants. Since melanoma is possibly caused by ultra-violet radiation from sunlight upon sensitive skin, the scarcity of this disease in north-west England will not surprise those who are familiar with the region! Britain also has the lowest liver cancer rates in the world, which is thought to be attributable to the scarcity of hepatitis B virus in Britain's cool climate and the high sanitation standards. It is possibly also due to the fact that little or no food is eaten after going mouldy, since the poison known as aflatoxin, present in many moulds, is thought partly to contribute, in association with hepatitis B virus, to the horrifying incidence of liver cancer in West Africa and many other hot, humid countries.

The challenge which has been facing physicians and scientists for many years has been to interpret these striking differences in cancer incidence in terms of their possible causes, and to come up with plausible means of removing those causes, so preventing cancer in many different countries. The fact that on the whole very little discussion about avoiding cancer takes place among doctors, and between doctors and their patients, should not be taken as any indication of a lack of knowledge or facts on this subject. When Professor Sir Richard Doll and his colleague at Oxford, Richard Peto, produced their landmark review *The Causes of Cancer* for the American Congressional Office of Technology Assessment in 1981, their first conclusion, namely that between 80 and 90% of all cancers could, in principle, be avoided, raised hardly an eyebrow in the medical profession on both sides of the Atlantic Ocean. This fact had been *suspected* for many a long year because it arises logically from the kind of disease-distribution findings I have mentioned. (The fact that Japanese men in Japan suffer 83 times greater an incidence of stomach cancer than women living in Iowa, USA, suggests strongly that 82 out of those 83 men could be saved from a painful death if only they knew what action to take.) But hard and fast proof about cancer causes is much harder to come by.

There is a widespread popular belief that tendencies which may predispose certain families or groups of people towards contracting cancers of various kinds can be inherited. If so, this would explain some of the differences between say, Japan's stomach cancer rate and that in the USA. But careful study of statistics concerning the importance of genetic factors in affecting people's cancer risks leaves the scientist with little option but to conclude that most of the difference must be explained by factors other than these. When, for example, stomach cancer rates among Japanese who have migrated to the United States are compared with those of similar ethnic backgrounds who stayed in Japan, it becomes clear that the migrants and their descendants sooner or later adopt the cancer risk levels which apply to the people in their *new* home.

There are a number of other popular myths about cancer which need to be exploded before people are likely to view cancer prevention as a real possibility. To begin with, people often think that cancer is on the increase these days. This is not true. Some cancers, such as lung cancer, *are* increasing, but others, notably stomach cancer, are becoming much less common. We tend now to talk about cancer more openly than in the past, which gives the impression that it is more prevalent, and also more people are now living to greater ages when the incidence of all diseases is high. But in each particular age bracket cancer overall is now slightly less common than earlier this century.

Another popular misconception is that cancer is infectious. It is not. You cannot catch the disease by visiting a patient suffering from it. Because this message is beginning to be understood more widely, people now admit more freely that relatives have cancer

Table III International changes in cancer death rates over a 25-year period (*c*. 1950 to *c*. 1975).

Country	Percentage change in death rate from cancer of: Stomach	Lung
Australia	− 53	+ 146
Austria	− 53	− 8
Chile	− 56	+ 38
Denmark	− 62	+ 87
England and Wales	− 49	+ 33
West Germany	− 50	+ 36
Ireland	− 54	+ 177
Israel	− 49	+ 58
Japan	− 37	+ 408
The Netherlands	− 60	+ 89
New Zealand	− 54	+ 137
Norway	− 59	+ 118
Scotland	− 46	+ 44
Switzerland	− 64	+ 72
United States	− 61	+ 148

(Adapted from *The Causes of Cancer* (OUP, 1981) by Doll and Peto.)

and this adds to the false impression I have already mentioned about cancer being on the increase.

The belief that all cancer is incurable is obviously untrue, as any of the thousands of former victims of Hodgkin's disease and other curable cancers will tell you. But that most forms of cancer are not easily cured *is* correct, especially the common ones: lung, breast, stomach and bowel. Even within this group there are some notable exceptions where people survive for many years and in whom the treatments, such as surgery, seem to be fully effective. I say *seem* to be, because the absolute proof of a cure is quite hard to show. Long-term survivors of the commonest forms of the disease, affecting mainly people of middle and old age, are in the minority among cancer victims – but they do exist, proving that cancer is not always a death warrant.

There is no convincing evidence that cancer is caused by stress, as is widely believed. The very idea that rich Western countries have the monopoly of stress and that this explains our high rates of particular cancers is, in my opinion, naïve and mistaken. To begin with, you cannot measure stress in any clear-cut way when one person's stress (such as driving, for example) is another person's idea of relaxation, and, secondly, it is ridiculous to suggest that life in modern cities is more stressful than life on the brink of starvation in the developing nations.

Pollution is another popular whipping boy, scapegoat for almost any national ill in the post-war era. Certainly, coal tar, some rarely used chemicals, asbestos dust and nuclear radiation (to name but four potential hazards connected with industry) can all cause cancer. But for most of us there is little chance of being exposed to these types of pollution and, in any case, most of them are now under such welcome legal control that we have little to fear at present about pollution causing cancer or any other disease to any great extent. The same reassurance can be given about food additives and chemicals used in farming. These are mostly consumed in minute quantities and are subjected to government limitations which should, it is hoped, reduce the chances of their causing cancer to very low levels.

So much for the myths about the causes of cancer. But what then are thought to be the main culprits? Although there is some doubt about all of the likely causes of cancer, certain factors are very firmly implicated: tobacco-smoking and long-term asbestos exposure, for example. A great deal of evidence is also gradually emerging which suggests that eating fatty foods helps cause the disease. At the same time there is a strong consensus of opinion that the eating of so-called dietary fibre and green and yellow leafy vegetables *protects* against a wide range of cancers. When foods which are thought to be protective against cancer are also known to be protective against heart disease, strokes and other ailments, then there is a very strong case (even in the absence of complete proof) for recommending that they should be included in what is now often called a 'prudent diet'. Alcohol, drugs, viruses and hormones should also be mentioned as being among the many suspected causes of cancer – although it is important to emphasise that smoking and eating habits seem to be more significant and more easily changed than most of these other factors.

So scientists are coming up with evidence about many of the

causes of cancer and this could now be communicated to the public. One obvious way of doing this would be via the family GP, but unfortunately doctors have little time or incentive to carry out preventive medicine for any disease, let alone cancer. In any case most general practitioners will lose touch with their patients during the long interval between exposure to a cancer risk factor and the disease developing. The family physician cannot look forward to the day, thirty years after advising precautions, when hundreds of grateful patients will be sending thanks and bottles of champagne to him or her for having ensured that they did not become exposed to factors which carry a one in 10, one in 20 or one in 100 chance of causing cancers. Even governments have little incentive to minimise the number of cancer deaths. Every citizen dying prematurely from cancer is a citizen fewer to be supported by social security in old age. The 'profit and loss account' does not even tip in the patient's favour if he or she receives medical treatment from the state. A dying cancer victim is unlikely to consume more national resources than a long-living senior citizen. For these, and for many other reasons, there has been national and individual inertia among those who have the power to implement cancer prevention in the communities of Britain, America and most of the industrialised countries.

It is against this back-cloth of global indifference to cancer causes and cancer prevention that a surprisingly large number of scientists have been working. After the studies which firmly established the connection between lung cancer and smoking, the most important of these scientists' findings are probably those related to diet and cancers of the stomach, bowel and rectum, and possibly also lung and breast. Something like a third of all cancers might be avoided by modifying the diet, according to Oxford scientists Doll and Peto, and although some other experts place more of the blame upon environmental factors, a great deal of consensus exists among cancer specialists about which foods to avoid and which foods to eat more of. Consensus medicine is being applied, with apparently high success, to preventing coronary heart disease. People are taking more exercise and eating fewer fat-containing foods for the sake of their coronary arteries. In the case of cancer the wave of public interest in disease prevention is only just beginning, and yet there are at least as many medical recommendations waiting to be communicated about cancer avoidance as have already been communicated about preventing heart disease.

It is worth pointing out, rather depressingly, that the simple knowledge of what causes a disease does not necessarily prevent its occurrence in the community anyway. Tobacco smoking has only declined moderately since the association with lung cancer was first proven. Yet individuals who smoke can be certain to reduce their risk of getting lung cancer by a factor of 10 – a very large risk reduction – by taking a very specific action: stopping smoking. What is largely absent in the community at present is a strong conviction that avoiding cancer is possible through such individual action. Part of the reason for this, as I have said, is that evidence about the appropriate actions to take has not been passed on clearly enough to the public at large. The question this book seeks to answer is: 'What are these actions?'

The detailed comparisons mentioned earlier between the pattern of life-styles in, say, Detroit and Ibadan and other places with strikingly different typical life-styles give scientists a great deal of *circumstantial* evidence about cancer causes and cancer avoidance. This cannot be taken at face value, of course, because scientific facts only emerge when the correct degree of emphasis or relevance is allocated to each observation. The way to achieve this is by probing the facts about human behaviour, diet, life-style, occupations, wealth, exposure to pollutants, exposure to climatic extremes and countless other variables with medical trials and studies. Such studies have been completed in hospitals and universities all over the world in order to investigate the particular properties of each factor thought to be a candidate for causing cancer. Each suspected factor then has to be isolated before its precise degree of importance can be estimated. The 'dietary fibre' content of foods consumed in Detroit, for example, is compared with the fibre content of foods consumed by the average citizen of Ibadan, both now and – even more important – during the previous decades. Also, the findings can be of no scientific significance whatsoever unless it is possible to find groups of people in the two cities whose life-styles, occupations, behaviour and other possible cancer-causing factors differ mainly in respect of the amount of fibre in the food. Such are the difficulties of achieving meaningful results from detailed scientific surveys. The complexity of the problem might seem insurmountable, yet clear insights *have* emerged which are judged to be scientifically valid because they are corroborated by further circumstantial evidence from other directions. In the case of fibre, for example, scientists have found that people who eat a fibrous, largely vegetarian diet have smaller quantities of bile acids in their stools (and therefore presumably in their bowels) than those who do not. Studies have shown that bile acids can, in some circumstances, be converted into substances which may cause cancer (see p. 62).

So, by looking at the scientific evidence it is possible to define a 'prudent' pattern of behaviour, life-style and diet which will hopefully help a person avoid most cancers. What is more, significant improvements in our cancer risk factors could be made without any traumatic or difficult adjustments. Protective factors could be added to our diet, for example, which would be eaten unnoticed along with other food. Even smokers who refuse to give up the tobacco habit can be helped in a number of ways as far as cancer prevention is concerned. (However, the risks of other smoking-related illnesses such as heart disease are unlikely to be reduced by the same factors as are believed to reduce the threat of lung and other smoking-related cancers.)

This 'prudent' life-style, which I have summarised in Chapter 8, is based on the groundswell of opinion which exists among many scientists who are tracking down the causes of cancers. Although some of them would like to wait for definite proof, many accept that some guidelines should be given now, as people will otherwise continue to follow patterns of behaviour already strongly suspected of helping to cause the disease. Although it is impossible to *guarantee* anybody freedom from cancer, these guidelines for prudent living are very likely to reduce your cancer risks quite significantly. By reading the evidence and comparing the ideal life-style with that currently available to most of us, you may come to the conclusion (as I have) that changes are needed to make it easier for us to follow patterns of living which are less likely to cause cancer. If, for example, your staff restaurant or works canteen serves chips every day rather than plain potatoes, you are justified in asking whether caterers should be given more education about the causes of disease than they are at present. If your doctor has never asked you if you smoke, you can feel justified in asking whether medical schools ought to include preventive medicine more often in the curricula than at present. These are just two of the many questions which I hope will arise from the facts presented in the rest of this book.

2 When living cells grow wild

The dream of cancer scientists the world over is to learn enough about the processes which cause cancer to be able to cure the disease. It has to be said right away that we are not anywhere near to such an understanding yet. The vital breakthrough which will solve the problem of cancer is not just around the corner, and may never even be made. But in the last few years some fascinating new insights into the mechanisms of cancer have been gained by scientists looking at the processes which happen in the cells of the human body. These do not promise a cure for cancer in the foreseeable future, but there is nevertheless more optimism now about the possibility of a practical pay-off from all the scientific hard work than there was a few years ago.

A tremendous international effort to conquer cancer has been made during the 1970s and early 1980s, with billions of dollars' worth of work going on in laboratories aimed at revealing the innermost secrets of the cancer cell. This work should perhaps be put into perspective in relation to the overall battle against the disease in which three broad strategies are being adopted. One of these is treatment, the second prevention, and the third biological research into the basic cancer cell mechanisms. In terms of practical benefit, medical treatment is at the 'sharp end', so to speak, affecting those who are already ill. That this can help such people by making them more comfortable is undeniable, but it is sadly true that most treatments currently available do not cure the disease.

Cancer prevention, through removing such cancer-causing substances as, for example, tobacco from our environment, is potentially the biggest contributor to the task of reducing human suffering from cancer in the near future. The third force in the battle against cancer, research into fundamental cell mechanisms, is currently contributing only a little to cure rates and to cancer prevention, but the hope is that one day knowledge about the basic science of the disease will lead to the answer.

Because the science of cancer is thought to hold out such promise for the distant future, there has been a mushrooming of interest in just about any aspect of the life-sciences which could possibly have a bearing on the problem, with both the Government and charities funding a plethora of branches of science which, to the uninitiated, may seem quite irrelevant to cancer. There are still too many unanswered questions for me to be able to give a full description of how cancer is formed in the body, but thanks to all this recent research into cancer and related sciences I can give a broad idea at least of the stages of understanding that scientists have reached.

The Cancer Cell

There is not much difference between a cancer cell and a normal cell of the body. Both consist of countless atoms joined together in complex and beautiful patterns. Both take oxygen and nutritious chemicals from the bloodstream and sustain living processes, including a capacity for self-reproduction. Both possess a pattern of genes, the DNA blueprint, which is unique to each person. But the DNA within each normal cell of the body contains the necessary information to reproduce an entire unique human being, whereas the DNA within a cancer cell is lacking in some way or may be distorted.

It is important to realise that when we talk about a cancer growth we are talking about living tissue which is similar to normal body tissues. It is so similar that our normal defences against illnesses and foreign bodies do not recognise the cancer cell as being 'alien'. Our bodies are equipped with whole regiments of different types of specials cells capable of doing battle with an invading organism, such as a microbe. These defences are so effective that even transplanted human tissues, such as a grafted kidney or heart from another person, are gradually recognised as being alien and, unless steps are taken to prevent this, attacked. This process is known as rejection. Unfortunately this does not

23

happen with cancer tumours. These are so similar to our own cells, being derived originally from them, that the regiments which comprise our immune systems are not 'ordered' to do battle with them.

There is a certain amount of justification for comparing a cancer cell to the cell of a human embryo shortly after fertilisation. Just like the embryonic human cell, which eventually grows into a fetus, the cancer cell possesses a complete set of genes which forms a blueprint from which a unique cancer tumour can grow and spread throughout the body. At the very early stage both human embryo and cancer cell have an ability to reproduce, and this seems to be unrestrained. By that I mean that the limitations which normally stop organs of the adult body from growing do not operate at this stage. When the early cancer cell or the early human embryo cell begin to multiply they both produce cells identical to the initial single cell which started off the whole process. But after a number of divisions, the offspring of such cells (both cancer and fetal cells) gradually become more different from each other, even though they continue to contain the same DNA blueprint. In the human fetus, this outward difference (called *differentiation*) is necessary in order to form different organs and parts of the body: skin, hair, liver and so on. In the cancer tumour such differentiation is not necessary for the survival of the growth. Although some tumours become quite 'differentiated', other cancer tumours remain relatively 'undifferentiated' throughout their existence. This is where the inherent character of the cancer growth and the human fetus can no longer be regarded as equivalent. Whereas most cells of a fetus gradually lose their initial urge to reproduce, forming specialised tissues from which to build a complete human being, cancer cells usually remain at a much more primitive stage of development. It is as if a cancer tumour were a fetus which never manages to reach the degree of maturity at which properly structured organs of the body become discernible. And because of this perpetual immaturity the cancer retains other characteristics which are not at all favourable as far as the victim is concerned whose body has been invaded by such a parasite. One is that the cancer retains an ability to grow without any form of regulation or restraint. This may not be a rapid growth, indeed some cancers grow very slowly, but it is nevertheless inherent in cancers that growth is potentially continuous, and this sheer competition with normal tissues is the reason why the disease is often fatal – indeed inevitably fatal in many cases. Another curious characteristic is the fact that cancers are potentially immortal. A type of cancer known as myeloma, for example, is widely grown in the laboratory for the purpose of manufacturing certain chemicals needed for tests such as blood-grouping. The original patient who donated his myeloma cells to a particular laboratory may have long since died, but the cancer cells which killed him will probably still be alive and well after many years in the laboratory test-tube. Ordinary tissues, even when grown in the test-tube, cannot survive indefinitely; they are strictly mortal.

The 'Rules' of Carcinogenesis

Although there are still many grey areas of knowledge, scientists *have* been able to establish some of the 'rules' which seem to apply to the development of cancer. These have been worked out as a result of painstaking experiments taking many months and years, in which the effects of different circumstances and various chemicals are tested for cancer-production in animals, especially mice.

One of the rules discovered is that carcinogenesis (cancer-formation) is almost certainly not an instant affair. People need to smoke for 20 years o more for there to be a reasonable likelihood of their getting lung cancer, and this gives a clue as to what might actually be happening to living cells when they 'grow wild' and turn cancerous. One reason for the delay is that cancer seems mostly to develop in a number of quite different stages, and each of the stages may be caused by a different factor or set of circumstances. The first stage is called *initiation*. This, and the later stages known as *promotion*, happen within a single cell. When all stages are complete, the cell has been fully converted into a cancer cell, which can multiply and eventually become a tumour. The fact that most cancer tumours originate from a single cell is fairly well established, because it is easy to test for 'family resemblance' in each of the cancer cells which form a particular tumour by establishing whether they each possess the same DNA or not.

The circumstances which initiate, or trigger, a cancer cell may be different from ones which promote the same cell. This is quite a hopeful state of affairs because it means that even when the first stage has taken place, it may still be possible to remove all risk of developing the actual disease of cancer by preventing further promotional stages from occurring. The work of a number of laboratories has established that certain chemicals, for example, act mainly as initiators of cancer, and others act mainly to promote an existing growth. Some circumstances both initiate *and* promote cancer, such as smoking which seems to be an initiator and promoter of lung cancer. (The two stages are very separate though and this seems partly to explain why it takes a number of years for this form of cancer to develop.) Experiments with mice have shown that a pure initiator, by itself, causes very few cancers when painted on the skins of mice, while a substance that only promotes initiated cells cannot cause a tumour. But if first the initiator and, secondly, the promoter are painted onto the mice skins, there is a good likelihood of cancer developing. I say 'likelihood', because it also seems that causing cancer is something of a hit-and-miss affair, rather like playing Russian Roulette.

Another characteristic of carcinogenesis is the so-called *latency period*. This is the period of time during which a tumour exists but cannot be detected. The period of latency is uncertain, for the obvious reason that if you cannot detect the tumour until it is quite large, you cannot establish exactly when it began its development. But the total length of time between the first triggering event and the appearance of the cancer *can* be accurately measured in some circumstances, such as by painting tars which are carcinogenic onto the skins of mice and waiting for cancers to form.

It has been suggested that the delay in the appearances of, say, lung cancer among smokers is largely because of the 'hit-and-miss' nature of the effect which smoke has. It may be, for example, that the first stage of carcinogenesis (initiation) may only happen after several years of smoking. This is possibly because the chance of individual smoke particles scoring a 'hit' and triggering off cancer is quite small, only increasing when a large number of cigarettes are smoked over a period of years. There may then be another delay, also dependent on pure chance, while the triggered cell waits for the next stage to happen (promotion). If there is more than one promotional stage in this overall pattern of cancer formation, the delay period could be even longer. Mesothelioma, for example, appears in asbestos workers an average of about 35 years after exposure to asbestos first took place. This may be because several promotional events have to occur to complete the development of the tumour.

The message to take home, then, is that the development of cancer is a hit-and-miss affair, subject to chance and the taking of risks. It cannot be stated that if you expose yourself to a particular thing you will inevitably develop the disease, but there is no doubt that the longer the exposure, the greater your chances of getting cancer. In some respects this is reassuring. Someone who smokes for five years and then quits will probably never develop cancer as a result of smoking: at least, all the evidence points in that direction. And occasional exposure to hazardous substances does not automatically confer the risk of cancer.

Dr Nicholas Wald of Oxford University describes the statistics of cancer formation as being rather like receiving penalty points for motoring offences. With up to a certain number you can continue to drive, but once you exceed that number you incur an automatic driving ban. With cancer this apparently means that if a smoker has already completed some of the stages in the development of lung cancer, then by stopping smoking he may avoid the final stage and never develop the disease.

Another important rule for any process which causes cancer seems to be that there is a clear relationship between the dose of, and period of exposure to, the carcinogenic factor and the likelihood of developing cancer. For example, although the chance of getting cancer from medical X-rays is very small, it is directly related to the number of X-ray examinations you have. If you have 40 X-ray examinations this will give you twice the risk of getting cancer as having only 20 examinations. (The risk would still be very small, however, and the medical benefits are always weighed against this tiny risk.) Similarly, if you smoke 40 cigarettes a day you run twice the risk of getting lung cancer compared with smoking 20 of the same type of cigarette. This is slightly complicated in the case of smoking by differences in smoking habits – less smoke may be inhaled when a large number of cigarettes are smoked – but the fact is still broadly speaking true that the more you smoke, the greater your chance of getting cancer. And it seems likely that this dose relationship is true for any carcinogenic factor – the greater the exposure, the higher the risk of cancer.

Reasons behind the rules

Can these known rules of carcinogenesis help us to understand what goes on at the most basic level in cells of the human body when cancer is formed? For example, what sort of disturbance can change a normal living cell of the body into a cancer cell? This is probably the area of greatest ignorance in the life sciences since there are lots of good ideas and no definite proof. One of the biggest difficulties in this whole field of study is that nobody has ever witnessed the event happening. Nobody has ever watched, under the microscope, a living cell being disturbed in some way and turning into a cancer cell. What is more nobody is ever likely to in the foreseeable future. The reason is that the body is built up from billions (actually about 10000 billion) living cells, any one of which could be the starting point of a cancer. Within each of these cells are countless atoms, which are themselves the basic building blocks of all things. The event which starts off the growth of a cancer tumour probably begins at the position of a small group of atoms within a single living cell. Looking for it would be *far* more difficult than finding a needle in a haystack!

Now that we must resign ourselves to the idea of never being able to see carcinogenesis in progress, what are the best *theories* about what happens? To explain these we enter the astonishing world of DNA biology. Every cell in our bodies contains this essential blueprint of life, and the odd thing is that each cell contains all of the information necessary for making an entire human being, even though obviously it does not do so. The fact that skin cells conveniently remain skin cells throughout our life, rather than growing into other tissues is all because of something called *gene expression*. Most of us are familiar with the idea that our inherited characteristics are contained in our genes, which are composed of DNA (so the DNA blueprint consists of a very large number of genes). But the question to ask about all of this is: 'Why are just a few of the genes "turned on" in each cell, while the rest remain dormant?' If your mother has blue eyes, you will then have a gene which is capable of giving you blue eyes too, but clearly this gene is not 'turned on', or *expressing* itself, if in fact you have brown eyes. This is commonly explained by saying that the gene for brown eyes, which you have inherited from, say, your father, is *dominant* and *suppresses* the activity of the gene for blue eyes which you have also inherited. (This is a familiar but oversimplified example. Genes for many other characteristics are also classified as either dominant or, the opposite, *recessive*.) One idea about the formation of a cancer tumour from an individual cell is that some of the genes (or perhaps only a single gene) in the cell's DNA, which are normally not expressed, may start to be expressed after the cell has been disturbed in some way. As most of the genes in the cell are quiescent and thus suppressed within any specialised tissue (being unwanted because they are appropriate only to the functioning of quite different types of tissue), it has been suggested that if one of these becomes activated it could derange the normal orderly behaviour of the cell. This may be what happens when some outside influence affects the cell in such a way that it turns into the initial cancer cell, which then, like the embryonic human fetus, begins to multiply, and eventually forms a tumour.

At this point in the story some exciting new developments in cancer science must be mentioned, because they have begun to clarify the picture of how cancer cells are formed so greatly that scientists are actually daring to hope that there could be a practical pay-off. A number of cancer-science research centres during the 1970s and 1980s have been searching for the particular part of the normal cell's DNA most likely to cause the unrestrained growth which is the characteristic of cancer cells and makes them different from most ordinary cells of the body. The findings of scientists in the USA such as Dr Mariano Barbacid (Bethesda) and Dr Robert Weinberg (Boston) have led to a belief that some individual genes in the DNA are responsible for turning normal human cells into cancerous ones. They have even managed to pinpoint a gene in human cancer cells now referred to as an oncogene (which simply means 'cancer gene'). Such genes, when 'switched on', give instructions to the cell to continue its growth and to reproduce itself, rather than not to do so, as it should in most normal mature human tissues. It is as if the cancer gene is putting back the clock, giving the cell the immature tendency to reproduce, just like the cells of a newly conceived fetus.

The scientists have found that cancer genes are normal genes possessed by every cell in the human body, which under normal conditions do not issue the harmful instructions to the cell which result in cancer developing. Why? This is where we come back to the concept of gene expression. A cancer gene may be normally suppressed and therefore inactive, like most of the genes in the cell which are not needed in any one specific type of tissue. But a disturbance could derange the cell in such a way as, for example, to affect the forces which hold this gene back from exerting its influence. This would explain something about why an outside disturbance is capable of triggering off cancer. DNA can be damaged by factors such as chemicals or radiation (known causes of cancer) and this could have the effect of lifting the restrictions which hold the cancer gene in check. The gene could thus become switched on instead of remaining switched off.

On its own this cancer gene theory, though attractive, does not help us to conquer cancer, but there are signs that for the first time it is giving the scientists a more complete view of what happens when 'living cells grow wild'. For example, in order to believe the idea that a particular gene causes cancer, you have to suggest how it might exert its action. Fortunately some of these mechanisms are becoming clear too. Dr Mike Waterfield at the Imperial Cancer Research Fund Laboratories in London has been studying the behaviour of genes in cancer for some time and in 1983 made two important discoveries. He found that a special 'growth factor', which scientists already knew to be involved in helping ordinary tissues to grow, happens to resemble very closely a type of protein which an oncogene has been found to manufacture. In the normal body the factor helps the processes which operate to repair wounds, and this discovery tempts people to speculate whether cancers are a form of wound-healing gone mad. The second discovery of the London team was that a so-called 'receptor' on the cell (which combines with yet another such 'growth factor') is made of proteins which also strongly resemble those made by an oncogene. What Dr Waterfield's research has shown is that a specific mechanism could exist, namely the combination of the chemical growth factor and the cell receptors, which might explain how parts of the cancer-forming process seems to operate under the control of genes in the central parts of living cells. The importance of this (as was pointed out to me by Dr Bob Downing of the Centre for Applied Microbiology and Research at Porton Down in England) is that it is now in theory possible to produce drugs which could either combat the growth factor or block up the receptors, and thus prevent cancer from spreading. This is far from being accomplished at the moment, but we can at least now look ahead to such possibilities; before the cancer gene concept was developed we had no such hope.

It is important to have reservations, however, about the prospects for stopping cancer in this way. To begin with there may be huge practical difficulties in developing such drugs. Secondly, most cancers have established many millions of cells in the body before they can be detected and by this stage it may be too late to benefit from such a treatment. So it is still important to look further into the processes of what might be happening within the cell to derange the DNA in such a way that the cancer genes are formed from normal genes and start to 'express' themselves and issue instructions, including ones which prompt the cell to make the growth factor.

Although it is known that certain drugs, chemicals and radiation can damage DNA and trigger off cancer, the precise sequence of events is still shrouded in mystery. It is by no means true that all processes which damage DNA, causing it to change (a process known as mutation), automatically cause cancer. But up to now it seems to be true that all processes which have been found to be carcinogenic certainly damage DNA (and are thus said to be mutagenic). So it has become very popular to test food additives, industrial and consumer products, in fact any new substance to which people may be exposed for any mutagenic action. When mutagenic action is discovered in a substance, it is excluded from human contact as far as possible. It is hoped that by this process mutagenic substances which are also carcinogenic are being excluded. There is no actual guarantee of this, however, because carcinogens may exist which are not mutagenic, and, in addition to this, the factors which affect the later stages of cancer development (the stages called promotion) may be quite different from those which affect the earlier initiation stages. It is not likely that promoters are even similar to initiators, and the fact that cigarette smoking apparently exerts both the initiation and the promotion of lung cancer is probably due to the fact that a large number of chemicals are found in the smoke, some of which may initiate, and others promote, the disease.

The scientific questions are a long way from being answered and there are still large gaps in our understanding of cancer-causing processes. On the one hand we know that certain factors cause cancer, and we think this is because they damage a cell's DNA and cause the initiation process to occur. But there is ignorance about the way in which this damage can cause parts of the DNA, such as the cancer genes, to be 'switched on' inappropriately, and we also know very little about the mechanisms within the living cell associated with promotion. Nevertheless important scientific tools have been invented by scientists such as Dr Bruce Ames of California who developed a test using the DNA from bacteria to detect mutagenic activity. It is a convenient and wondrous fact of nature that bacterial DNA is so similar to human DNA that we can safely assume that things which cause mutations in the cells of microbes will also cause them in human cells. The Ames Test for mutagenicity is now one of our standard safeguards for excluding mutagens from the environment, although whether or not they would actually have caused cancer in humans we shall never know.

The pattern is emerging

The fact that cancer genes are now largely thought to explain the process of carcinogenesis is a very big step towards understanding why cancer can be caused by a variety of means. The idea that an outside influence of some type is necessary to switch on a cancer gene is leading scientists to search for factors which are capable of influencing DNA when they come into contact with a cell. Because living cells are encased in a membrane we can assume that the only outside influences capable of causing cancer are the ones which can penetrate this. Viruses are one such type of agent which can enter the living cell and actually live inside it, even incorporating their own DNA into the cell's DNA. And viruses are among those agents suspected of causing cancer. Chemicals can also cross the membrane and reach the DNA so it is not surprising that the chemicals in cigarette smoke can do this, just as can the chemicals in special carcinogenic tars when painted onto the skins of mice. Radiation is another agent which can pass right through the cell and can certainly cause mutations in DNA, and it is definitely known that radiation can cause a wide variety of cancers. But a much more difficult thing to understand is how certain body chemicals such as hormones are involved in triggering or promoting cancer and how other changes in our body chemistry, perhaps caused by food, influence our chances of getting the disease. For example, a growing body of evidence is implicating factors such as fat in our diet as helping to cause certain cancers, but we are a long way from fully explaining why.

It would be satisfying to be able to say definitely how particular things cause cancer, and that this is known because the scientific knowledge about the inner workings of the living cell has proved this or that. No such definite final statement can be made. But I do not think this should prevent us from advising people about how to avoid cancer. Modern scientists always talk in terms of the limits of their knowledge rather than certainties, and some think that it would be better to wait for all the questions to be resolved before going public and advising people how to avoid this disease. I take the opposite view, namely that to hold back from giving to the public the knowledge we now have, incomplete

33

though it may be, would be to do everybody a disservice. Every one of us has to make decisions each day about how to behave even if this is only deciding on whether to walk or take the bus, whether to eat potatoes or chips, whether to start smoking, or whether to take that extra alcoholic drink. The scientific knowledge I shall present in the remaining chapters is intended to give you at least some idea of the possible consequences of such decisions, and to have more confidence in your ability to avoid what may prove to be an unnecessary illness.

3 Hazardous habits, hazardous jobs

Although vast sums of money have been spent on laboratory investigations into the microscopic behaviour of living tissues and cancer cells, this basic science has not yet yielded much practical pay-off in terms of solving the cancer problem. But there is another approach that has already turned up many clues which I mentioned in Chapter 1, namely the making of comparisions between different groups of people. This is done in order to examine the ways in which cancer incidence varies from place to place, from time to time, and between one sector of the community and another (especially between one type of worker and another). These comparisons can never in themselves give absolute proof about the causes of cancer, but they give very powerful evidence. For example, the fact that mesothelioma is a very rare type of lung tumour in most of the population but is one of the commonest cancers among asbestos workers does not in itself prove that asbestos causes mesothelioma. But it gives very strong suggestive evidence that it does. The fact that bowel and breast cancers are less common in countries where less fat is eaten *suggests* that dietary fat has something to do with the development of these cancers. But because both breast and bowel cancer are very widespread in many countries where hugely varying patterns of diet are found, the association of fat-eating with these cancers can be regarded only as a clue, not even as strong evidence, about the causes of these cancers. The findings must be corroborated by a mass of other scientific evidence (which I shall describe in Chapter 4) before a warning against eating fat can be given. A great many such clues about the causes of cancer are continually being uncovered. This is because increasing numbers of medical scientists and statisticians have now focused their attention upon the important question of finding suspected cancer causes by making detailed comparisons of life-styles of different communities.

It is as though the entire world were a laboratory, but with experiments being conducted voluntarily by different people: eating various foods, doing different jobs, having different habits. The voluntary experiments going on all around us give scientists the opportunity of reaping a rich harvest of information which has already helped piece together many of the parts of the jig-saw puzzle about cancer. It would be wrong to suggest that this is as yet complete, but it would also be unreasonable to hold back from drawing interpretations, especially as some of the evidence about the causes of the commonest cancers is very strong.

The classic case of a type of cancer of which the cause has been accurately and conclusively tracked down by making such detailed life-style comparisons is lung cancer. The great popularity of smoking began in Britain as long ago as the turn of the century, when cigarettes became more available as an alternative to cigars and pipe tobacco. Ironically, the decisive British medical investigation which finally proved that smoking causes lung cancer was already being planned after the Second World War when the Chancellor of the Exchequer, Stafford Cripps, suggested that we should all, on grounds of economy, smoke our cigarettes down to the butts.

In the 1940s, opinion-leaders ranging from politicians to film-makers and advertisers could be forgiven for failing to suspect that smoking might kill people. Today there should be no forgiveness. The medical warnings are very dire indeed, and there can be little doubt (as emphasised recently by the Royal College of Physicians) that governments are falling far short of their responsibilities. Some have gone so far as to describe the situation as the 'tobacco scandal', because there is now the clearest possible evidence that smoking has a one in four chance of killing anybody who takes up the habit.

Britain has the highest lung cancer rates in the world. The disease increased among men a staggering 50-fold between 1911 and 1970, an epidemic rise which followed, after a delay of about 20 years, the rise in popularity of cigarette smoking. The classic idea of a 'latent period' found in laboratory animals was clearly obvious from these voluntary 'human experiments' too.

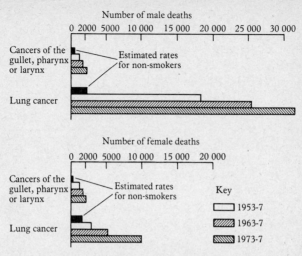

Fig 3 Number of deaths caused by lung cancer and cancers of the gullet, pharynx and larynx in the USA over three five-year periods.
(Reproduced from *The Causes of Cancer* by Doll and Peto (OUP, 1981).)

Although Britain leads the world in both smoking and lung cancer, America is catching up rapidly. What is even more horrifying is the fact that women in Britain, America (*see Fig 3*), and many other countries are now suffering a growing epidemic of lung cancer, which began 20 years or so after cigarette smoking became thoroughly 'acceptable' for women (namely, after the Second World War). In the 1920s and 1930s only the more daring, sophisticated, or outrageous women were willing to be seen smoking. But the war provided wages for women and released female inhibitions about the habit, helped not a little by movies which portrayed smoking as an activity in which the most glamorous women (and men) engaged.

How the case against smoking was proven

Although it was suspected that the increase in lung cancer was linked to the adoption of a habit whereby smoke was regularly drawn into the lungs, sadly in medicine it is usually thought necessary to be certain of the facts before recommending people to change their ways. This was the situation which faced Dr Richard Doll of the Medical Research Council and Professor Austin Bradford Hill of the London School of Hygiene and Tropical Medicine after the war when they set out to find enough evidence to incriminate or exonerate smoking as a cause of lung cancer. It took them two years to complete even the first part of their investigation; the dotting of i's and crossing of t's is still being done today.

Because the United Kingdom is a world leader in both smoking and lung cancer, it is not surprising that the massive investigation to work out whether the two were linked was carried out in Britain. But in the United States there was also plenty of concern about the lung cancer problem (even though that country was, up until then, blessed with a fairly large proportion of non-smokers) and in the late 1940s Dr Ernst Wynder in the Washington University School of Medicine investigated the issue with the help of the leading surgeon, Ewart Graham. Since that time many studies of large numbers of smokers have been carried out which have underlined most of the messages first urgently spelt out by these classic early investigations.

In Britain Doll and Hill decided to interview a large number of patients suffering from lung cancer. In all statistical matters, the larger the numbers, the more accurate the conclusions, and so by interviewing nearly 1500 lung cancer patients in several different cities the scientists were able to build up an impressive databank of information. An important part of the method of study was the way in which each cancer patient was matched with another patient in the same hospital at the same time, and of similar age and the same sex, but who was not suffering from lung cancer. The two scientists used the matched subjects not suffering from lung cancer as a comparison group. In this way they hoped to pinpoint the distinguishing characteristics of lung cancer patients.

Using a 'matched control group' turned out to be vitally important, because at that time about nine men out of every ten in Britain were smokers, so the simple finding that there were a large number of smokers among the lung cancer patients would have meant nothing. By making a detailed comparison with the 'control group', however, it was possible to make a very comprehensive range of remarkable discoveries about the relationship between smoking and lung cancer. Doll and Hill asked both the lung cancer victims and the matched 'control' subjects questions about their past and present smoking habits – how many cigarettes, cigars or ounces of tobacco they smoked each day; whether they inhaled or just puffed; smoked plain or filter-tipped cigarettes; used a holder or a cigarette lighter; at what age they started smoking; and how much tobacco or how many cigarettes they had smoked at various earlier times in their lives.

There were only 100 or so women lung cancer patients among the group of 1500, and it was tempting at that time to imagine that women might be relatively immune to lung cancer. Doll and Hill correctly suggested, however, that this was likely to be related to the fact that smoking had not been sufficiently popular among women for long enough to cause the disease. Today we can see only too clearly how the popularity of smoking among women has inevitably caused lung cancer in them too.

The results: very few non-smokers get lung cancer

One of the astonishing facts to come out of the study by Doll and Hill was that there were only seven life-long non-smokers among the 1357 lung cancer victims. Among the same number of 'matched controls' there were 61 life-long non-smokers. (The scientists defined a non-smoker as anybody who had not smoked as much as one cigarette a day for a whole year.) So, although smoking was extremely popular even among the subjects who did not have lung cancer, the difference in the numbers of *life-long* non-smokers in the two groups was very large. Also there were far more heavy smokers in the lung cancer group than in the control group.

To inhale or not to inhale?

Among the lighter smokers there was not much difference in the lung cancer rates between those who inhaled the smoke and those who just puffed their cigarettes. But, curiously, among the heavy smokers, inhaling the smoke deeply into the lungs was actually slightly less likely to result in lung cancer, though the overall risk of the disease was still very high.

Cigarettes versus pipes or cigars

Pipe and cigar smokers did not seem to get lung cancer nearly so frequently as cigarette smokers, but to this day it is not quite clear whether changing from cigarettes to a pipe or cigars will give a cigarette smoker any protection. *Life-long* pipe or cigar smokers, however, do not seem to face the same cancer risks as life-long cigarette smokers.

Cigarette holders and filter-tips

The study seemed to show that using a cigarette holder was less risky than smoking cigarettes without a holder, and filter-tipped cigarettes (just becoming popular at the time the study began) also seemed to be less hazardous than plain cigarettes.

Female smokers

As far as the women lung cancer victims were concerned, there was a greater proportion (40 out of 108) who claimed to be life-long non-smokers than among the men, but the risks were just as clearly related to heavy smoking.

Length of exposure

It was found that the risk of getting lung cancer increased with every cigarette smoked. The more people smoked each day, the more likely they were to get lung cancer, and the longer they continued to smoke the greater the risk, with about 20 years of smoking being necessary before the disease was first detected. People who started to smoke at a very young age were more likely to get lung cancer, and the small number of people who had contracted lung cancer in their thirties or early forties were generally those who had started smoking very young and had thus smoked enough cigarettes to develop the disease.

What about the butt?

According to a later study which Doll and Hill (together with their colleagues Gray and Parr) published in 1959, the length of cigarette ends discarded by smokers does seem to make a difference to their chances of getting the disease. The investigators had wanted to explain the fact that Americans who smoked the same number of cigarettes for similar periods of time as British smokers seemed to have a lower risk of getting lung cancer. In this study they compared the length of cigarette ends discarded by Americans and Britons and discovered that the average American butt was 31 millimetres long as compared with only 19 millimetres average in Britain.

Smoking is like 'Russian Roulette'

Most of the facts which Doll and Hill discovered can be explained if the risk of getting lung cancer from smoking is largely a hit and miss affair, like Russian Roulette. Some smokers who don't get the disease *may* be protected to some extent by their 'constitution', by being inherently more resistant to the carcinogenic action of tobacco smoke. But for most people it is pure chance which dictates whether a cancer tumour will start to grow or not. This is exactly the same phenomenon as is observed in animals exposed to carcinogenic substances in the laboratory. Not all of a group of identical mice will get cancer, and nobody can predict in advance which animals will remain free of the disease. It seems to be a matter of pure chance, although if the carcinogen is powerful enough and applied for a sufficiently long time, then all the mice will develop tumours.

No smoker should therefore imagine that he or she is immune from cancer. The evidence suggests that the ones who have not already developed the disease are simply lucky, rather than actually resistant to it. The longer they continue to smoke, the more they are pushing their luck.

Lower tar yields cause less cancer

Studies about smoking and lung cancer are still being carried out in many laboratories, for we certainly do not have all the answers yet. It is fairly clear, however, that it is the sticky residue which can be collected from cigarette smoke – the so-called tar – which contains the cancer-causing agent or agents among the hundreds of different chemicals in this sinister cocktail. In 1981, Sir Richard Doll (who had been knighted in 1971 for his achievements in this field) published a study jointly with Dr Nicholas Wald of Oxford and Mr Graham Copeland in London which documented the changes in tar yields of cigarettes during the previous 50 years. Packets of cigarettes dating from as early as the 1930s and covering most of the years up until the 1980s were donated by a large number of people so that the scientists could analyse them to find out whether tar yields of cigarettes had altered over the years.

They discovered that modern cigarettes yield less tar than those manufactured before the Second World War. This was due not only to the introduction of filter-tipped cigarettes after the war, but also to changes in the formulation of tobaccos used for making the cigarettes. The three scientists stated that the 50% decrease in tar yields since 1934 seemed very likely to be responsible for the reduction now reported in the numbers of people who die from lung cancer. During the same period of time, nicotine and carbon monoxide levels in cigarettes have not changed very much, so it seems to be the tar which is responsible for causing lung cancer, rather than these other candidates. So reducing tar yields does seem to be a way of making cigarettes a little safer as far as causing lung cancer is concerned, although no such hopes are held out that this would also make them less likely to cause other conditions such as heart disease, bronchitis, emphysema and high blood pressure.

A second classic study

Richard Peto, who is now working in collaboration with Sir Richard Doll at Oxford, is very concerned about the fact that most people in Britain and other countries are continuing to smoke cigarettes despite the fully documented evidence which proves that moderate to heavy smoking carries a very high health risk. Smokers are not only dying from lung cancer but are also contracting other serious diseases, namely heart disease, bronchitis, and several other types of cancer – gullet, mouth, throat, and possibly pancreas, bladder and rectum. Doll and Peto published the results of a massive survey in 1976 which Doll had begun in 1951 together with Professor Austin Hill by sending out question-naires to 34000 male British doctors asking them about their smoking habits. The doctors have been followed up ever since, and there have been further questionnaires asking them about changes in smoking habits. As doctors in this group die, the causes of death are noted and compared with each doctor's use of tobacco. This gives the scientists a unique opportunity to re-test all of the previous ideas and findings about the health conse-quences of tobacco and cigarette smoking. By 1971 10000 of these doctors had died and Peto and Doll were able to analyse the information.

Doctors are a particularly interesting group because they are among the most likely people in the country to understand the implications of the findings which have been made about the rela-tionship between cigarette smoking and lung cancer. More than half of the doctors who reported that they smoked in 1951 gave up the habit after this time. When they replied to the later question-naires they gave full details about any changes in their smoking habits, complete with dates, and this made it possible to calculate more precisely what the health benefits of stopping smoking were likely to be.

The study showed once again the frightening statistic that about one heavy smoker in every five can expect to get lung cancer (with many of the others dying prematurely from other tobacco-related diseases). But when the effect of giving up smoking was examined, there was a very encouraging finding: the risk of get-ting lung cancer starts to fall quite drastically from about five years after quitting smoking. Ten years after stopping the risk is only a third as high as if the person had continued to smoke, and 15 years after quitting (assuming he is still alive) the ex-smoker's chances of getting lung cancer are not much different from those of a life-long non-smoker. Even people who have smoked for several decades can cut their risks of getting cancer by stopping smoking. There is no 'point of no return'; quite the contrary, in fact – every extra cigarette adds to the smoker's chances of developing lung cancer (not to mention the other smoking-related diseases), so quitting makes sense at any time.

Encourage the non-smoking fashion

Not enough is being done to educate smokers about the benefits of stopping the habit, according to Richard Peto, who says that even doctors are not doing as much as they could to advise patients not to smoke. He claims that when doctors explain fully the risks of smoking, the evidence shows that one smoker in 20 will give up the habit permanently. In national terms this means that 2000 people each year could be spared from dying early of lung cancer, and probably more could be saved from experiencing the other dangerous consequences of smoking. With a note of exasperation in his voice, Peto asserts that if only the smoking problem could be taken more seriously by doctors and governments, a great deal of human misery could be saved. The study of British doctors has shown that entire groups of people can be persuaded to give up the habit if given the right information and it does seem that certain social classes are giving up smoking. In the upper echelons of society the message about smoking and health is getting through. If only this could also filter through to other social groups there is a chance that it could become socially undesirable in *all* walks of life to smoke cigarettes. The fashion of not smoking could catch on!

In the meantime Richard Peto thinks that to save the lives of present-day smokers who will not give up it is important to look into ways of making cigarettes safer than they have been in the past. The study which Nicholas Wald and his colleagues conducted about the tar yields of different cigarettes from 1934 up until the present day shows that improvements have already been made by manufacturers, and it might be logical to try to push these improvements to the limit. One way, says Peto, is to follow up the suggestion made a number of years ago by Dr Michael Russell of the Addiction Research Unit at the Institute of Psychiatry in London; namely that the ideal cigarette should contain a lot of nicotine and as little of everything else (including tar) as possible. This is a controversial idea because doctors do not yet agree about which of the compounds in tobacco smoke are the main causes of heart disease, which kills more people than lung cancer. But Peto thinks that nicotine is probably not very hazardous – indeed Dr Wald recently discovered that pipe smokers seem to have lower risks of heart disease than cigarette smokers, even though they absorb the same amount of nicotine. So a case can be made out for boosting the nicotine yields of cigarettes so that smokers will inhale less smoke to get the same amount of nicotine. This idea arises, of course, because nicotine is an addictive substance and is one of the things in smoke which a truly addicted smoker needs to get. If a smoker cannot give up the addiction, then boosting the nicotine yield might reduce the number of cigarettes he smokes and, at the same time, his intake of tar.

To lend strength to some of these ideas, Michael Russell and his colleagues have carried out a number of studies in which other sources of nicotine are used to help smokers give up tobacco smoking. Nicotine-impregnated chewing gum, snuff and nicotine nasal sprays all seemed to help people to give up smoking, and did not seem to be as addictive, but other studies have not found these alternative sources of nicotine to be so much of a help.

Risk to women confirmed

The survey of male British doctors begun in 1951 was accompanied by an exactly similar survey of female British doctors, and in 1980 (after a long period of mathematical analysis) Peto and Doll published their findings – that women seem to face exactly the same risks from smoking as men. There is no protection by any factor related to their sex, and the fact that lung cancer was previously quite rare in women is shown, as in other studies, to be the result only of the fact that until fairly recently not many women smoked, and those that did smoked in a different way.

Even today lung cancer is still three times more common in men than women. Although smoking became quite socially acceptable for women in the 1940s it has taken until now for the epidemic of lung cancer among women to build up. Before very long it looks as though lung cancer will overtake breast cancer as the most frequently diagnosed form of the disease in women. Alarmingly, school-girls seem to take up the habit of smoking more often than school-boys. This may be because they think that it helps to keep their weight under control, but it is a shortsighted and unwise action. There is no hard scientific evidence to back up the idea that smoking helps you to stay slim.

Exporting smoking problems to other countries

Not satisfied with the dubious honour of being the leading country in the world for both smoking and lung cancer, Britain is contributing to the introduction of smoking into Third World countries which are seen as a promising new market for tobacco products. An editorial in the *British Medical Journal* in May 1979 revealed that the British Government made grants during the 1970s of £30 million to the British tobacco industry. During the same period of time only £2 million was spent on health education to discourage people from smoking. When questioned about this surprising fact, Mr Roland Moyle, then Minister of State for Health, said in a parliamentary reply that jobs in certain development areas were one reason for certain grants being given to the tobacco industry. Another reason was that: '. . . a considerable part of the production will be exported, bringing significant benefits to our balance of payments'. From this we can assume that the priorities of a healthy British balance of payments are considered in Whitehall to be more important than healthy human lives in the countries to which we export tobacco products, including now the Third World.

A World Health Organisation expert committee on smoking control published a report in 1979 entitled *Controlling the Smoking Epidemic*. The committee members considered that: 'The international tobacco industry's irresponsible behaviour and its massive advertising and promotional campaigns are direct causes of a substantial number of unnecessary deaths'. But large industries cannot be expected to react to suspected health problems unless there is genuine public concern, and one of the big problems about the hazards of smoking is that there is no such outcry. The dangers of this particular cancer cause *have* been communicated to the public and some steps have been taken to help protect people from smoking. But most of us now seem to accept that no further progress will take place and that our children will be exposed to cigarette advertising and peer-pressure in favour of smoking just as we were in the past. Some young people fortunate enough to be able to resist these pressures may avoid the addiction. But should we wash our hands of the threat which faces the others?

Governments have nothing to lose and everything to gain from leaving tobacco legislation and health education campaigning as they are today. Currently smokers contribute enormous tax revenues and obligingly die at younger ages from diseases which do not usually require expensive hospital treatment for long periods of time. If a country such as Britain abandoned smoking overnight it is doubtful whether the National Health Service could cope with the extra care that would be needed for old people surviving in the future who would have died from heart disease, cancer, or strokes had they not given up smoking. It is doubtful too whether the Government could finance the pensions and social security payments which would be needed without heavy taxation on workers, who would be the minority in a population where longevity had greatly increased. On the other hand, it would surely be possible for the economic strategists to plan to take advantage of the better health which would be enjoyed by such people. The costs *could* be balanced in the right direction.

Is other people's smoke dangerous?

Although cigarette smoke is a nuisance to non-smokers in restaurants, offices, pubs, cinemas and other public places, there has not yet been much evidence to indicate whether this could be a danger to their health or not. In Japan Dr Takeshi Hirayama recently noted that non-smoking wives of heavy smokers were found to be at a higher risk of getting lung cancer than similar women whose husbands did not smoke. And in 1983 Dr Pelayo Correa of the Louisiana State University in New Orleans, USA, reported on a study which he and his colleagues had conducted of such 'passive smoking'. This showed that non-smokers married to heavy smokers had an increased risk of lung cancer, and so did people whose mothers smoked. Yet smoking by fathers didn't affect the risk of lung cancer among the offspring. The investigators do not suggest that we now know everything there is to know about the dangers of passive smoking, but there are certainly enough worries about it to justify a good deal of further action, such as prohibiting smoking in many public places and gradually restricting it to an activity which is only tolerated among consenting adults in private!

Encourage quitting

Although smoking is addictive, there are encouraging findings from a number of studies aimed at finding out the best way of helping people to quit the habit. One of these was reported in 1983 in the *British Medical Journal*. The Australian *Quit for Life* programme carried out in New South Wales consisted of a scientifically planned campaign in which two test towns were studied. In one there was extensive media publicity given to the dangers of smoking and other health issues. In the other no such campaign was mounted. The result was that 16% of young men quit smoking in the town where the publicity campaign was mounted and a 5% decline occurred in the 'control' town used for comparison. (Some reduction in smoking is taking place all over Australia as a result of other sources of information about smoking not related to this special programme. The control town happened by co-incidence to receive a wave of publicity about smoking dangers during the test period.)

This Australian study took two years and proves that young people can be influenced to refrain from smoking. Backed up by national resolve and government support there is no reason why smoking should not lose its appeal. It would be quite simple to give smoking the bad image it deserves – as the murderer of millions of innocent people. When governments see fit to consider this an expedient course of action we could see a shift away from tobacco smoking happen quite quickly.

Many smokers would like to give up the habit but are embarrassed to do so when most of their friends or colleagues smoke. Most people find it difficult to do something different from those around them. But if they received emotional support, for example from a television campaign which featured successful and glamourous people who do not smoke, many might feel able to cope with the difficulties of giving up a habit which had become second nature to them.

Cancer in the work-place

An important category of people who are making it possible for scientists to study the causes of cancer are those who are exposed to factors at work which are suspected of being carcinogenic. There is a link here with our 'volunteer' smokers, because one of the leading types of occupational cancer is lung cancer. It is not surprising that some of the fumes and dusts concerned in industrial and mining jobs have the ability to damage the lungs. Other parts of the body can be protected by clothes, but it has not been until quite recent times that most workers have been adequately protected by face masks and other equipment from the dust and fumes which can cause lung cancer.

Asbestos

Asbestos is another substance now known to cause the types of lung cancer found in smokers and it also causes the form of the disease know as mesothelioma. Among some groups of asbestos workers as many as one in five have died from lung cancer, and the danger is not only from long-term exposure. Nine months' work in an asbestos factory in the United States was shown to double the risk of lung cancer, and men who worked temporarily in shipyards during the Second World War have also been found to be at a higher than average risk of developing this disease. Most of the deaths from lung cancer do not happen until 30 or more years after exposure to asbestos, so it is predicted that there will be many more deaths in the future as a result of past exposure to asbestos dust before guidelines and laws were passed to protect workers.

The effect of both smoking and working in the asbestos industry is very dangerous indeed. The two cancer hazards do not merely add together, but actually multiply each other's risks. Heavy smokers who are not exposed to asbestos have about 20 times the risk of getting lung cancer that non-smokers have. But in one study it was found that a group of heavy smokers who worked with asbestos in America experienced *90 times* the risk of contracting lung cancer. It is interesting, however, that the asbestos-related cancer—mesothelioma—is not any more likely to develop in smokers than in non-smokers. This presumably means that this form of cancer is caused specifically by asbestos, and not tobacco smoke.

There is no doubt that the dangers of working with asbestos are being reduced, and for non-smokers they may be quite small today in most advanced countries. But the dangers to smokers are still far from negligible, and the danger to workers in the asbestos industries of countries where regulations are unfortunately not so advanced as in places such as Europe and America are still as large as ever.

When asbestos is not disturbed it is harmless because the dust fibres are not released into the air and so cannot be inhaled. But the current fears about asbestos have created a new danger. Recently there has been a great deal of activity within the building industries of many countries to remove asbestos from old buildings. It is difficult to devise regulations and guidelines to control such work and guarantee that workers and public alike will not be exposed to asbestos fibres from the way in which it is carried out. For a number of years while the work is being done there may therefore be an added risk from asbestos dust being released into the air – a risk which has arisen as a direct result of panic over asbestos dangers. In general, it is better not to disturb intact asbestos.

The asbestos saga illustrates vividly how cancer hazards can come from unsuspected directions, and that such hazards can take many years to be detected in the community, by which time it is probably too late to prevent cancer developing in many of the people who have already been exposed. As new industries are set up it is important to bear in mind the possibility that some of the substances used may cause cancer and to test them to ensure they are safe. As a result there will in future be greater protection for workers from dangerous dust and fumes, so there is less risk of workers being exposed to a hazard as severe as asbestos. But the risk of cancer hazards at work is something about which nobody should be complacent.

Uranium mining

Lung cancer is also more common among uranium miners, such as those in the Colorado plateau of the United States. This is because the miners inhale the radioactive gas called radon during their work and all sources of atomic radiation, including X-rays, are capable of causing cancer. The miners have an extra risk which is equivalent to smoking more than 40 cigarettes a day, and those who smoke are at an even greater risk of contracting the disease.

Other cancer hazards at work

Cancer hazards at work are, of course, crucially important to the groups of workers in the particular industries where these arise, but they actually account for only a small fraction of human cancers (between 2 and 8%, according to some experts). Over the years governments and industry have become aware of the possibility that many different substances can cause the disease and a great deal of improvement in working conditions has been made during the twentieth century to remove many such hazards. Hopefully, therefore, exposure to many of the well known industrial causes of cancer has now been considerably reduced. These include the dyestuff industry, where some of the chemicals used were found to cause bladder cancer among workers. Coal-burning industries – particularly involving the production of coke – have in the past exposed workers to a variety of fumes, including gases called polycyclic aromatic hydrocarbons, which cause cancer in animals and have been associated with lung cancer in some workers. Wood and leather dusts cause cancers which begin in the nose and sinuses among employees in the wood-working and shoe-making industries. The manufacture of chromium and nickel products can cause lung cancer, and the refining of mineral oils in the petroleum industry has been found to cause skin cancer, which also affects machinists who use these oils for cutting and grinding metals. Asbestos causes a wide range of cancers in addition to lung cancer and the type of mesothelioma which affects the lung. The lining of the abdomen, for example, can also develop mesothelioma as a result of asbestos exposure, and

Table IV: Workers at risk

(NB Some of the broad occupational categories given here include, of course, many people who have never worked with the causative agent listed.)

OCCUPATION	PROBABLE AGENTS	SITE AFFECTED
Asbestos workers (miners, textile manufacturers, insulation workers, etc.)	Asbestos	Lung, pleura, peritoneum (also possibly stomach, large bowel, gullet)
Asphalters	Polycyclic hydrocarbons★★	Skin, lung
Aluminium refiners	Polycyclic hydrocarbons★★	Lung
Arsenical pesticide manufacturers	Arsenic★	Skin, lung
Coal gas manufacturers	⎰ Polycyclic hydrocarbons★★ ⎱ Some aromatic amines	Skin, lung / Bladder
Chromate manufacturers	Chromium★	Lung
Cadmium workers	Cadmium★	Prostate
Copper smelters	Arsenic★	Skin, lung
Cobalt smelters	Arsenic★	Skin, lung
Dye manufacturers	Some aromatic amines	Bladder
Farmers/Open-air workers generally	Ultraviolet light in sunlight	Skin
Gold miners	Arsenic★	Skin, lung
Glue workers†	Benzene	Marrow (especially erythroleukaemia)

Hardwood furniture manufacture	Unknown	Nasal sinuses
Isopropyl alcohol manufacturers Ion-exchange resin manufacturers	Isopropyl oil Bischloromethyl ether	Nasal sinuses Lung
Leather workers Luminizers	Unknown Ionizing radiations	Nasal sinuses Bone
Miners (mainly uranium, some others)	Ionizing radiations	Lung
Nickel refiners	Nickel*	Nasal sinuses, lung
Poison gas manufacturers PVC manufacturers Pigment manufacturers	Mustard gas Vinyl chloride Chromium*	Larynx, lung Liver (angiosarcoma) Lung
Roofers Radiologists and radiographers Rubber workers	Polycyclic hydrocarbons** Ionizing radiations Some aromatic amines	Skin, lung Marrow (all sites) Bladder
Seamen	Ultraviolet light in sunlight	Skin
Varnish workers†	Benzene	Marrow (especially erythroleukaemia)

* Only certain compounds or oxidation states of these substances have been found to be carcinogenic. ** Contained in certain tars, oils and soot as products of incomplete combustion. † Also other workers who use benzene-based solvents. (Adapted from *The Causes of Cancer* (OUP, 1981) by Doll and Peto.)

cancers of the gullet, throat, stomach and large bowel have all been linked with this substance, giving it the dubious distinction of being the cause of the widest range of industrial cancers from a known single agent. Vinyl chloride, a substance which is made into that universally useful plastic PVC (polyvinyl chloride) is the cause of cancers of the liver and possibly of the brain and lung among past workers in the plastics industry.

Learning from experience

So altogether the list of known industrial carcinogens is now quite long (*see Table IV*). It is tragic that people who have worked with such substances in the past have been exposed to these cancer hazards, but at least their suffering has resulted in these causes being firmly identified and cancer scientists have been able to derive important knowledge from this about carcinogenic substances and how cancer is formed. As a result, the industries I have mentioned are now a good deal safer and, as long as vigilance is maintained, should become even safer in the future.

The information gained from people who have died as a result of industrial cancers has been compared with findings from the type of laboratory experiments mentioned in Chapter 2 and some important facts are emerging. To begin with it has been confirmed that with most of the substances that cause cancer among workers there is a latent period between exposure to the carcinogen and diagnosis of cancer. This can be as short as one year in some cases, but may be as long as 50 years. In the case of asbestos, for example, the average latent period is about 35 years before mesothelioma is detected. Although there appears to be no known safe level of exposure to a carcinogen, it has been found in animal experiments that the more of a carcinogen you are exposed to, the greater your chances of getting cancer. The age at which exposure takes place is the most reliable means of predicting when a cancer is likely to be detected. Just as in the animal experiments, it seems to be nothing to do with old age itself. The cancers are more likely to appear in older people simply because they are more likely to have had a long exposure to the cancer-causing substance.

Present day knowledge about work-related cancers makes it clear that long-term exposure is the most dangerous, and that each exposure to a carcinogenic substance adds to the risk that cancer will actually develop. Just as in smoking cigarettes, there is the element of Russian Roulette about this kind of risk. Many workers will never get cancer, and the ones who docannot be predicted on the basis of any inherent susceptibility or inborn tendency to be 'cancer prone'. It seems mainly to be a matter of pure luck, unless the exposure is so high that almost every worker develops the disease. The only known case of this was when 16 men who actually distilled the chemical beta naphthylamine in the dyestuff industry all developed bladder cancer.

Cancers caused by hazards at work underline once again the message that cancer is not inevitable, and that it has causes which can be avoided. Although these may form only a small fraction of current cancer cases, they illustrate the point that it is worth seeking out the more common causes of cancers (which now seem to be related to aspects of every-day living) in the hope that these may then be eliminated from our way of life.

4 Eating can seriously damage your health

A moment's thought tells us that in the twentieth-century Western world eating has become far more than a necessity. More people than ever before no longer eat merely in order to live, but live largely for the joy of eating. It has been elevated to the position of one of the top pleasures in our pleasure-seeking society. The growth of 'food worship' is aided and abetted by modern industry which provides us with an un-ending variety of delicious gastronomic experiences, ranging from hamburgers and fries to chocolate-coated sugar–glucose bars. How unfortunate it is that some of the most popular foods in the West seem to help cause some of our commonest types of cancer.

One of the relevations contained in the Doll/Peto report to the US Government in 1981 on *The Causes of Cancer* was that, in America, a third of all cases of cancer are probably caused by eating habits. This was a necessarily conservative estimate because of uncertainties which have yet to be solved, and the importance of food in causing this disease may eventually turn out to be far greater, not only in America, but in most other countries. On the brighter side, as well as foods which may *cause* cancer, there are others which may prove to protect us against it.

There is very little argument among cancer scientists about the suggestion that a large proportion of the world's cancer cases are the result of a variety of eating habits. But when it comes to saying precisely what it is about our food which gives us cancer, or protects against the disease, there is far less certainty. Absolute proof has not been found either for beneficial foods or for any of the suspected culprits, but the circumstantial evidence in many cases is very strong. In the words of Professor Sir Richard Doll: 'The problem is to decide when the evidence is strong enough to justify action to modify the diet'.

Evolution and the modern diet

It no longer comes as a surprise to most people to be told that modern eating habits may cause disease. Our bodies were 'designed' before the era of well stocked supermarkets and fast-food restaurants, and a huge appetite was then necessary for survival. Darwin's theory of the survival of the fittest suggests that our large appetites are the natural result of evolving over millions of years in the 'hunter-gatherer' societies of pre-historic times. Those who did not eat a great deal on the far fewer occasions when plentiful food was available did not survive. But now that the lean times are over (for a quarter of the world's population in the industrialised countries at least) our big appetites are no longer appropriate.

So the discrepancy between the primeval appetite and the present day bodily requirements of *homo sedens* (sedentary modern man) gives us an inborn tendency to overeat. This would not be so bad if it were not for the sorts of food which are most easily available to us. Today's Western diet is highly refined and concentrated, containing high levels of meat and fats, which long ago our ancestors could not get in regular, large amounts, and refined sugar and white flour which were not then available.

Even before scientific evidence connecting food and cancer (and, for that matter, food and other 'Western diseases' such as heart disease) had been produced, we might have at least suspected that the great changes in our eating habits, which have, for the masses, only been possible since the Industrial Revolution, could be a source of danger. The change from running and labouring to catch, grow or gather food, to simply buying it from a shop, combined with the switch from unprocessed wholegrain foods to a highly processed and concentrated meat and sugar-rich diet seems intuitively to pose possible hazards. At the same time it would be quite wrong to suppose that all change is likely to be harmful as far as cancer is concerned. What emerges from a look at the world cancer pattern is that while many of our *former* eating habits seem to have protected us against getting certain cancers, some of our *modern* eating habits almost certainly protect us from other types of cancer. Bowel cancer, for example, is very common in countries eating a typical Western diet and may be avoided by changes to eating patterns which were common before the Industrial Revolution. But stomach cancer is becoming less common all over the Western world, and has become quite rare in the United States – the country which consumes the most typically 'Western' diet.

The art of improving your diet to avoid cancer, then, is to combine the best of the old with the best of the new, and not simply to make generalisations. The only way to do this is to look at the scientific evidence which has been accumulated so far.

Western diseases and lack of fibre

A tremendous stir of excitement took place in the world of the cancer detectives in 1969 when Denis Burkitt (known for his discovery of the cancer called Burkitt's Lymphoma – a rare disease mainly affecting children in Africa) published an article in the medical journal *The Lancet* under the title 'Related Disease – Related Cause'. Having spent a great deal of his working life as a surgeon in Uganda, he was struck by the absence of appendicitis, bowel polyps (small growths), diverticular disease and cancer of the large bowel and rectum in traditional, rural African communities – diseases which are only too familiar in twentieth-century Britain and America. His article suggested that these 'Western diseases' result perhaps from one single cause present in the rich countries, but not present in the Third World. The difference which he thought to be important was 'dietary fibre' – the part of our food which is not digested by the body, but which passes all the way through the gut until it reaches the large bowel (the final part of the intestines) where it is digested by bacteria.

Burkitt took the opportunity of building upon the ideas of a pioneer of modern dietary thinking, Surgeon Captain T. L. Cleave of the Royal Navy, who in the 1950s suggested that refined foods, especially sugar and white flour, cause a wide range of Western diseases. These foods contain less fibre than natural, unprocessed foods such as wholegrain cereals and vegetables, and, according to Cleave, they make it possible for us to consume too much carbohydrate. This is because refined carbohydrate foods go down easily into the gut and are absorbed quickly by the body. Unprocessed foods contain indigestible cell walls which impede the absorption of any carbohydrate (energy-yielding) constituents, so at the root of Cleave's ideas was the belief that if you get rid of the natural fibre and feed people on the refined carbohydrate (which is exactly what sugar and white flour consist of) you run the risk of consuming far more than is good for you. Fibre acts as a natural protective barrier, slowing down the rate of food absorption by the body and giving the feeling of satiety after a meal which discourages further eating. It also helps with the physical activity of the intestines since bulk, or roughage as it is sometimes called, helps the food to pass easily through the gut.

Cleave was already working on these ideas in 1941 when he gave sailors on the battleship *King George V* daily rations of bran to help with constipation, but since that time people have often made the mistake of thinking that bran is the only form of fibre of any importance and that adding it to a Western diet will solve all our problems. In fact, according to Cleave, the important thing is not to interfere with nature in the first place, i.e. not to separate natural fibre from other food constituents. His work paved the way for Denis Burkitt's theories, studies and observations which now give us the clear message that dietary fibre, especially in natural wholefoods, may have a powerful protective effect against bowel cancer.

Cleave's ideas about Western diet and modern illnesses such as heart disease, diabetes and bowel cancer, came both from his observations while travelling the world with the Royal Navy and also from vigorous correspondence with scientists from many different countries in the 1950s and 1960s which kept him abreast of the latest findings of others working on related topics. He put forward the idea that today we can satisfy our craving for sweetness by eating refined sugar, but if we had to eat unprocessed fruits to derive the same amount of sweetness we would have to consume a great deal of dietary fibre along with the natural sugar in fruit. We would thus eat less carbohydrate because the bulk of the fruit would limit the amount we could consume. So in modern times it is easy to overconsume, eating far more than would have been possible during the years of our evolution as the human species.

Among the many Western diseases which Cleave attributed to the eating of refined (fibre-depleted) foods was bowel cancer, and Denis Burkitt homed in on this when he wrote his article in *The Lancet* in 1969, combining Cleave's logic with his own brilliant interpretation and observations gained from working in Third World countries like Uganda. Burkitt's proposal that fibre is the crucial factor in protecting us from disease is in harmony with Cleave's ideas that foods should be eaten in their natural form. One reason for the neglect of dietary fibre at this time was because fibre was defined as the substance which remained after a food had been boiled first in acid and then in alkali (caustic solution) in the laboratory – a drastic treatment, which left only a tiny residue of undissolved material from most foods. (This is now called 'crude fibre'.) In the human gut, however, foods do not get such drastic treatment and very much more residue is left, which passes into the large bowel where it is digested by bacteria and forms the stools. 'Dietary fibre' – the undigested residue *in the gut* – is present in much larger quantities than the 'crude' fibre of the old definition, and it is quite clear that since dietary fibre is the only type of food residue likely to have important health consequences in the human gut, it is very much more relevant to discussions about diet and disease.

It is quite remarkable that appendicitis was at one time thought to be caused by food residues getting trapped in the appendix and a low-fibre diet was therefore thought to be less likely to cause the disease. In fact the reverse is true, according to the logic of T. L. Cleave and the studies of Denis Burkitt, so high fibre or wholefood diets are now recommended to avoid appendicitis. Likewise, during the last 20 years we have seen the recommended diets for diverticular disease reversed. Until the late 1960s this painful bowel disease was treated with low-fibre foods. But it is now generally accepted that fibre-rich foods, such as wholemeal bread, cereals, fruits and bran, not only help relieve the symptoms, but can also stop it from developing in the first instance. Both Cleave and Burkitt thought that it was no coincidence that appendicitis, diverticular disease and bowel cancer are common in the same countries, and felt that they were probably caused by the same factor, which they also thought to be responsible for constipation, piles, ulcerative colitis, diabetes and even heart disease. Cleave had named sugar and white flour as the culprits, but Burkitt came to the conclusion that lack of dietary fibre was the cause.

Since then, more information about the distribution of bowel and other cancers throughout the world has become available, and there is still no major contradiction of Cleave and Burkitt's fundamental idea that in places where people eat foods in their natural, unprocessed form (which automatically means that they eat foods rich in fibre), the incidence of bowel cancer and other Western diseases is low.

One notable exception to this is Japan, which has a low bowel cancer rate even though the Japanese eat no more fibre than the British, who suffer far more from this disease. But this does not rule out the idea that foods in their natural fibre-rich form protect against bowel cancer. It simply suggests that something as yet unidentified is responsible for *causing* bowel cancer and that this may be absent from Japanese diets, so the protection of fibre is not required in Japan. It may not be a co-incidence that the Japanese eat very little in the way of fatty foods, and neither do Africans, who also contract little bowel cancer. But more of that later.

How fibre may work

In his reports of the late 1960s and early 1970s Burkitt presented various attractive scientific ideas about why a lack of fibre in the diet could allow bowel cancer to develop. He suggested that dietary fibre could have the effect of diluting any cancer-causing substances in the food passing through the bowels. This would happen because of the extra bulk provided by the fibre. As well as this, he carried out experiments to find out how rapidly food passes through the digestive tract. He gave people small plastic pellets to eat with their food, which could then be followed by X-ray as they passed through the body or which were collected from stool samples after defaecation. This meant he could monitor the length of time taken for food to pass from mouth to anus. He discovered that a high-fibre diet gives a rapid 'transit' through the digestive tract and so suggested that this would reduce the length of time during which any cancer-causing agent would be in contact with the wall of the intestines. It would thus make it less likely that such an agent could exert its effect. It has also been suggested that because fibre causes certain bacteria naturally present in the gut to diminish in numbers and other strains of bacteria to proliferate, this could affect the 'environment' in the gut and perhaps make cancer less likely.

Since Burkitt's report in 1969, interest in dietary fibre has been intense and investigations are in progress in many different centres all over the world where his and Cleave's ideas are being put to the test. Dr Michael Hill, for example, of the Bacterial Metabolism Research Laboratory in North London (now at Porton Down, near Salisbury) has examined the idea that bacteria in the gut might form potentially cancer-causing substances which result in bowel cancer. He and his colleagues found that individuals from countries with a high incidence of bowel cancer and where little dietary fibre is eaten had higher concentrations of substances called 'bile acids' in their stools than people from places with a low incidence.

These substances, which help with the digestion of fats in the bowel, are not thought to be capable of causing cancer in their natural state, but when they are changed (by a process called dehydrogenation), they form a chemical which is thought to be capable of starting off cancer tumours. When looking at patients who actually had bowel cancer, Hill and his colleagues also found higher bile acid concentrations in their stools. As well as this, another distinguishing feature usually present in greater amounts in the stools of such patients than in the stools of patients suffering from other diseases was a particular type of bacterium known to be capable of changing the otherwise harmless bile acids into carcinogenic substances.

The picture looked complete, and Hill's idea about bacteria being involved in the cancer-forming process was well illustrated by this work. The only way to achieve final proof that high levels of bile acids and the particular strain of bacterium (evocatively named *Clostridium para-putrificium*) actually cause cancer is to take stool samples from large numbers of healthy individuals, store them, wait for subjects to develop bowel cancer, and then test the stools from those people for bile acids and the clostridia.

Michael Hill, together with Dr Tudor Hart in Wales and Dr Tom Meade and colleagues at the Northwick Park Hospital near London, are in the process of doing this, but it will take many years before the answers are finally known.

Fibre differences and British cancer rates

Important further confirmation of the protective role of dietary fibre against bowel cancer came from a group at the Dunn Nutrition Unit in Cambridge, England, in the 1970s. Sheila Bingham there says that the problem with comparing traditional African diets with Western ones is that as well as eating a great deal more fibre, the rural African also eats very little fat and animal protein, so any of these three factors could account for the rarity of bowel cancer in Africa as compared with the West. She thinks there are good reasons for looking into the effects of eating fibre, citing her colleague John Cummings' view that fibre is not an inert substance. Although it is not digested by the gut, when it reaches the final part of the bowel, the large bowel, it is consumed by bacteria. These incorporate water and the unrefined carbohydrates from the fibre into their cellular structure and thus form a great deal of bulk in the large bowel. This explains why the rural African's stools have greater weight and faster transit times through the bowel, as was noticed by Burkitt. It all fits in well with the idea that fibre helps dilute any cancer-causing substances which reach the large bowel (which is, incidentally, the part of the bowel most usually affected by cancer) and that the processes by which bacteria could otherwise help produce cancer-causing substances might otherwise be diverted into forming large bulky stools.

Cummings and his colleagues developed these theories from studying healthy volunteers in Cambridge under accurate, scientific conditions. But how well do they compare to real life? Another of the Cambridge group, Dr David Southgate, pioneered accurate methods for measuring the amount of dietary fibre in various foods, and this made it possible for Sheila Bingham and Dr Rhys Williams to make a comparison of different parts of Great Britain in terms of the amount of fibre eaten and the rates of bowel cancer. In Scotland bowel cancer is a more common cause of death than in the South East of England, and it was found that fibre there was less popular. But it was one type of fibre in particular that seemed to make most of the difference: the so-called pentose fraction, most commonly found in wholegrain cereals. On the face of it this seemed to be straightforward confirmation of the idea that bran can protect against bowel cancer. It was also found that in the areas with the highest rates of bowel cancer, including Scotland, people ate green vegetables less often than in places such as South East England where bowel cancer rates are lower.

Bingham realised that other things in the diet might make a difference to cancer rates and perhaps cloud the issue, so she and her colleagues carried out an investigation into the amount of whole-grain cereal fibre eaten in relation to the incidence of bowel cancer in Scandinavia. It was known that rural Finns suffer from only one third the rates of colon cancer compared with Danes living in Copenhagen, and Bingham and her colleagues did chemical analyses of the diets of a random selection of Danes and Finns from these two different types of area. It turned out that the rural Finns ate more of all types of fibre, including cereal bran, mainly from eating more rye bread than the urban Danes. So this study confirmed the finding in Britain that more fibre is eaten in places where bowel cancer is less common. All in all, the Cambridge work is yet more confirmation of the ideas originally put forward by Burkitt and Cleave that foods in their natural, unprocessed form are likely to help protect against bowel cancer. As Sheila Bingham points out, until more is discovered about dietary fibre it seems sensible to eat more of it to be on the safe side, particularly wholegrain cereal and vegetables. So the ideas put forward by Cleave and Burkitt have been endorsed by others, and it is significant that their recommendations have already withstood more than 15 years of thorough scientific scrutiny, from Cambridge and elsewhere.

One of the more recent studies in this area has been carried out in Toronto, Canada. Dr Tony Miller there has constructed a study of bowel cancer patients and a carefully selected group of similar people not suffering from cancer, for comparison purposes. He was not actually able to find any difference between the two groups in the amount of fibre eaten, but he does say that this does not necessarily rule out the idea that fibre protects against bowel cancer. He explains that in a modern country such as Canada most people tend to choose from a fairly similar range of foods, and it is simply not common to find large differences in the amount of fibre eaten from one person to another. In contrast, rural Africans eat much more fibre than Canadians or other Westerners, so Dr Miller concludes that we may need to make a major alteration to our fibre intake to change significantly the numbers of people suffering from bowel cancer.

'Majority verdict' on fibre

However good the theory, and however persuasive the circumstantial evidence, the final proof about diet and cancer can only come from very large-scale studies. Our diet needs to be investigated over a long period of time among various groups of people, who then need to be followed up to discover whether certain eating habits have increased their risk of contracting certain cancers or not. This takes many decades of dedicated work and is already being started in Japan, Britain, America and parts of continental Europe. Neither is the continent of Africa (the fountain of a good many modern nutritional ideas) being neglected in this detective work. The final proof of ideas put forward by Burkitt and others about fibre will take a long time to be documented, and even the best ideas may be shown to be mistaken. But most nutritionists now regard the indigestible component of foods, the fibre, as being of great importance to health generally. The consensus of opinion among nutritionists and cancer epidemiologists is that Burkitt is probably right, and that very little harm and a great deal of good could come from recommending people to eat more fibre. The real problem, which I shall look at in Chapter 8, is to find convenient ways of doing this in our modern society.

Dying off the fat of the land

It seems to be ingrained in Western culture that eating foods containing fat is the equivalent of living the 'good life'. Expressions such as 'living off the fat of the land' neatly sum up our attitude, and most people's favourite dishes, ranging from ice-cream to pork sausages, all contain a great deal of fat. Because fat is so popular in the West, food manufacturers take every opportunity of adding it to foods to 'improve' the flavour. When you look at a recipe for a British favourite such as shortcake it is astonishing to realise that half the weight of this biscuit is butter or margarine. Fast-food restaurants seem to specialise in fatty foods: hamburgers inevitably contain fat in the meat, and these are usually eaten with french fries and may even be washed down with a creamy milk-shake. The more traditional fish and chips is hardly less rich in fat, especially as the doughy batter on the fish soaks up the fat during frying.

Is this amount of fat in our food safe? The answer now seems to be a firm 'no'. Not only are fatty foods convincingly suspected of helping cause heart disease, but a major American report now recommends that Americans (and other Westerners eating similar foods) should reduce their fat intake to avoid cancer. The report was compiled by an authoritative panel of experts who looked at a wide range of scientific evidence on behalf of the American National Research Council and their report, called *Diet, Nutrition and Cancer*, was published in 1982. The evidence examined concerned a variety of possible foods which could cause cancer. Dietary fibre was an important category which came under scrutiny, and the recommendations made agree with those of pioneers such as Denis Burkitt. But the evidence the experts summarised about the way that fat, in particular, seems to be involved in causing cancer is startling, especially in view of the very great popularity of this food ingredient in the West.

I do not want to give the impression that all of the lines of evidence are fully proven; diet is a complicated subject and it is not always possible to be certain about cause and effect. But in spite of these difficulties, the evidence is so strong that, as someone who has been trained and worked as a scientist, I am personally quite convinced that fat is dangerous and very likely to be the cause of some of the commonest cancers in Western countries.

Fat and breast cancer

One of the most important pieces of evidence is simply the fact that certain types of cancer are much more common in countries where fatty foods are most popular. A number of different experts have drawn up comparisons with the amount of fat-containing foods eaten in different countries and the incidence of cancers of the breast. Dr Bruce Armstrong and Sir Richard Doll published one such study in 1975, and a different investigation was also reported by Dr Ken Carroll in Canada in the same year. It is clear from these that places such as Britain, the Netherlands and the United States suffer from very high rates of breast cancer, whereas Japan and Thailand, where traditional foods contain much less fat, have very low rates of this disease (*see Fig 4*).

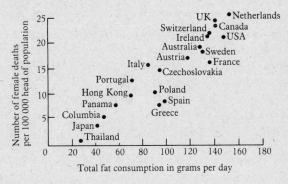

Fig 4 Chart showing the total daily consumption of fat and the death rate from breast cancer in various countries.
(Redrawn from a paper by K. K. Carroll in the journal *Cancer Research* Vol. 35 (1975).)

Of course, this kind of overall evidence is not enough on its own to incriminate fat as a definite cause of breast or other cancers, so a number of scientists have looked into what breast cancer patients eat and compared this with the diets of similar women who are not suffering from breast cancer. Dr Roland Phillips did this among a community of Seventh Day Adventists in California in 1975. These are a particularly interesting group of people because, for religious reasons, they mostly adhere to a diet which avoids meat; they also discourage smoking and drinking. Because they eat very little meat they consume less fat than most Westerners, on the whole (although dairy produce is not actually forbidden by their religion). But this sect is of particular value to scientists for another reason: they are a stable community and they keep good records of health information. Because of this Roland Phillips was able to carry out a study which initially seemed to show that breast cancer patients had eaten more fat during their lives than the comparison group of women. On continuing the studies, however, he has not been able to prove such a link. In Canada Dr Tony Miller carried out a similar study of breast cancer patients in 1978, and he too found a relationship between the eating of fatty foods and the later development of breast cancer. Miller's study did not show a very strong link, but it was difficult to be sure that the diet reported by the women at the time of the study was necessarily the most relevant. It is widely thought that diet early in life has the most important effect on future breast cancer risks, and so this makes scientific investigation more difficult because people cannot easily remember what foods they ate as children and young adults.

On the island of Hawaii there are fascinating opportunities for looking at different groups of people with various cultures: native Hawaiians and immigrant Japanese and Americans, for example. These different groups eat different foods, and some eat mixtures of foods which are a blend of traditional foods from different places. Dr Lawrence Kolonel was able to look into the consequences of different diets among the various peoples of the Hawaiian 'melting pot' and he also found, in 1981, that the groups of women who ate more fatty foods were more likely to get breast cancer. There will always be arguments about whether this evidence means that fat actually *causes* breast cancer, or whether both breast cancer and the eating of fatty foods are related to some other factor shared by high-risk groups as yet to be identified. Nevertheless, at present the most plausible explanation is that fatty foods *are* a cause of this form of cancer.

Fat implicated in other cancers

A number of different lines of evidence seem to prove that fatty foods cause other types of cancer too. Dr Kolonel's surveys on Hawaii found that cancer of the prostate (which is very common in old men in the West) was related to eating more fat. In 1975

Armstrong and Doll confirmed by looking at national cancer statistics in different countries that there was a relationship between average per capita fat intake and cancer of the body of the womb, a suggestion originally made by A. J. Lee. Very strong evidence exists too which suggests that bowel cancer is caused by fat. (This is clearly a different matter from the discovery that dietary fibre seems to *protect against* bowel cancer.) Armstrong and Doll, for example, mention in their report that countries where the most fat is eaten generally suffer from the highest rates of bowel cancer.

When you look at studies of fat intake in particular countries, however, it is not always easy to show up this relationship. In the study by Sheila Bingham of Cambridge, UK, in which inhabitants of the rural region in Finland called Kuopio were compared with a group of town-dwellers from Copenhagen, Denmark, the Finns were found to experience much lower rates of bowel cancer than the Danish group, even though their fat intake was found to be the same. It was noted, as I have already mentioned, that in Kuopio the population ate a great deal more dietary fibre than the people in Copenhagen. This primarily seems to uphold the theory already discussed that fibre has a protective effect where bowel cancer is concerned, but it does not actually rule out the possibility that the Danes could as easily lower their bowel cancer rates by reducing their fat intake as by increasing their consumption of fibre.

The reason that scientists are becoming more and more convinced that fat is a major culprit in causing cancers of the bowel and womb, as well as the breast, is that, quite apart from the statistical evidence, there are also some very good scientific explanations as to how this could happen. In the case of breast cancer, for example, fatty tissues help to generate the female hormone, oestrogen, in the body which, it is already known, can help cause breast tumours to develop (see Chapter 7). Dr F. de Waard in Holland has advanced this as an explanation of why typically short, slim Japanese women suffer from less breast cancer than taller, more weighty Dutch ladies. Bowel cancer is another case where a scientific explanation has been put forward, namely that food can affect the internal environment of the gut (and the types and quantities of bacteria which live there). This has led to the theory that fat could be converted into substances called bile acids in the bowel, and that these could be transformed into cancer-causing substances by the microbes in the gut. As I mentioned earlier in connection with fibre, a lot of evidence suggests that people with high concentrations of bile acids in their stools have the greatest risk of getting bowel cancer, but the research on this is not yet complete. As with the evidence about breast cancer and fat, these incomplete pieces of evidence need to be judged in the light of the comparisons between the rates of cancer in different countries. Any single piece of the evidence could not be taken as absolute proof in itself, but collectively the facts should serve to discourage us all from eating an excess of fat, and to suggest that it is high time Western people looked into the many different ways in which they could radically reduce their intake.

Animal experiments as long ago as 1942 were already implicating fat as a cause of various cancers. Dr A. Tannenbaum carried out a study in America at that time in which the calorie content of food given to laboratory mice was considerably reduced. The main purpose of a whole series of experiments he performed was to find out whether underfeeding the animals generally resulted in any variation in cancer rates and I shall be looking at this aspect of diet next, but one of the findings to emerge from his work was that reducing fat on its own did result in fewer cancers developing in the mice.

The National Research Council's report of 1982 on *Diet, Nutrition and Cancer* presented three lines of evidence incriminating fat as a cause of cancer, especially cancer of the breast, bowel and prostate. Firstly, comparisons between different countries suggest that the more fat eaten in a particular place, the more the people there suffer from these cancers. Secondly, comparison-controlled surveys of patients have pointed to the same conclusion (despite the difficulties entailed in establishing accurately what people eat and used to eat in the past). Thirdly, laboratory experiments on animals have produced similar results. Only the fine details still remain to be added.

Finally, fatty foods are a very concentrated source of calories and energy and are easily absorbed by the body. Because of this we easily run the risk of overeating if we eat a lot of fatty foods.

Obesity, which is partly caused by overeating, is related to a number of different cancers, so this suggests yet again that it is a good idea to cut down on fats.

Overeating – the Western temptation

The body of evidence which suggests that some foods (such as fat) cause cancer, and others (such as dietary fibre) prevent it has to be viewed along with evidence that it is also the sheer *quantity* of food we eat which may contribute to the incidence of this disease. Most people would agree that in general in the West we have ample opportunity to overeat and that this is one factor (though not the only one) which can lead to obesity. For some years a connection between being overweight and contracting cancer has been suspected, and records kept by insurance companies about the physical condition of their clients does seem to bear this out. Such companies have known for a long time that being overweight puts a person at a higher risk of dying from heart disease – a 50% higher risk if you are about a third heavier than average for your height. Then in 1960 the Metropolitan Life Insurance Company of New York published their finding that people who are 20% overweight also ran a higher than average risk of getting particular cancers.

In Britain, Armstrong and Doll's 1975 report comparing the risks of contracting cancer in different countries showed that the risks for all types of cancer in each age group were highest in the countries where the most food is eaten (all types of food: calories, fat and meat protein) and lowest in countries where national statistics showed that the least food is eaten.

In New York in 1979 Edward Lew and Lawrence Garfinkel of the American Cancer Society reported the results of a massive study of the differences in the numbers of deaths from cancer and other causes among a cross-section of the general public. They found that people who are 40% overweight (and who therefore can be classified as 'obese') had double the risk of dying at any particular age than people of average weight, and that extra deaths from cancer accounted for a significant amount of this risk.

In particular, men who were between 30 and 40% heavier

than their ideal weight (who could be described as 'mildly obese') were found more often to die from cancer of the prostate and the large bowel. Their risk was up by a factor of between a third and two thirds. Women were at an even higher risk of dying of cancer as a result of being overweight. Even being as little as 10% over-weight conferred a more than 50% extra risk of getting cancer of the gall bladder or biliary passages in such women. In addition the breast cancer risk was 50% up in women who were more than about 40% overweight (this is categorised as obese). And there was also found to be an extra risk in even mildly overweight women of getting cancers of various parts of the womb and of the ovaries.

Of course these statistics do not mean that *all* overweight people will get cancer; most never will. But it is nevertheless true that more overweight people develop the disease than those of average weight. This is obviously one further incentive, if an incentive is needed, for anybody who needs to take slimming a little more seriously. It is important to emphasise that these are not big risks: smoking five cigarettes a day would be a much larger risk (though for different types of cancer) than being a little over-weight. But among the many possible risks there are, extra body weight is one further small risk which could be avoided.

Eat up for a shorter life

The fact that cancers are slightly more common among people who are overweight gives extra emphasis to the suggestion which has been made by some scientists that the sheer quantity of food we eat can affect our cancer risks. As a theory this could never be put to the test on humans, of course, but scientists have tested the idea on animals.

As long ago as 1940 Dr Tannenbaum in America first looked into the way in which cancer rates in mice are affected by changes in diet. Astonishingly he found that cutting down their food rations drastically reduced the numbers of cancers suffered by groups of laboratory mice. Most scientific laboratories allow mice unrestricted access to food, which seems both logical and humane. But this is very different from the pattern of access to food which animals experience in the wild. Laboratory mice are notoriously prone to cancer, and usually live only for about two years. But when Tannenbaum reduced their intake of all food by about half the mice lived on average for about three years and hardly any of them suffered from cancer! What is more, the laboratory mice that were given unlimited amounts of food to eat became fat and sluggish, whereas the underfed mice were fit, sleek and active. It is hard therefore to escape the conclusion that restricting the mice's diet improved the general quality as well as the length of their lives, in addition to preventing the development of cancer.

The next step was to find out whether it made any difference to the mice if one particular type of food were restricted rather than another. In the 1940s Tannenbaum, and other scientists fascinated by this work, tried restricting each food component in turn: fat, carbohydrate, protein and so on. By varying the diet in only one aspect in any one study it was hoped that the most important dietary causes of cancer might be identified.

It was found that reducing the intake of energy-giving foods (both fats and carbohydrates) had the biggest effect in reducing the incidence of cancer. This was found both in animals which were allowed to live normally without any special treatment, and also among those given substances to eat which were known to cause cancer. Calorie-restricted diets diminished the tendency of mice to develop cancers even when specific attempts were made to induce these by feeding them with carcinogens. The same was true when cancer-causing substances were painted onto the skins of mice: restricting their calorie intake delayed or prevented skin cancer from forming.

Evidence from animal experiments has, of course, to be looked at with a critical eye. It is not always so that something found to be true in animals will also hold true for humans since we have very different genetic qualities and live in ways which are far removed from the environment of mice in cages. But nevertheless there are also great similarities between humans and mice, and a great many medical problems are solved first by trying them out on animals before subjecting humans to something new. In the field of developing new drugs and new methods of surgery this has paid off handsomely and for this reason alone we would do well to heed the warnings from evidence about causes of cancer arising from such tests.

The scientific findings reported from many different centres of research on the prevention of cancer in animals by restricting different foods were summarised in 1979 by Dr David Jose of Melbourne, Australia. The work of Tannenbaum has been repeated and refined in many centres with the overall finding that restriction of carbohydrates and fats together brings a big reduction in naturally occurring *and* artificially induced cancers. When animals are given a sufficiently large dose of a cancer-causing substance the effect of underfeeding can be overcome and tumours will be produced, but even so these usually take longer to develop than in animals who are given more food and subjected to the same amount of the carcinogen. If only one of the two energy-giving constituents of food (fat or carbohydrate) is restricted there is a smaller reduction in the numbers of cancers, and if you give mice extra fat to make up for a deficiency of carbohydrate this makes them just as likely to get cancer as mice who are given the normal mixture of food in unlimited quantities.

This is exactly comparable with the information we have about how cancers form in humans. Scientists now believe that carcinogens can cause cancer in anybody who is exposed for a sufficiently long time to a sufficiently large dose. It seems to be true that all smokers could get lung cancer if they smoked enough cigarettes for a sufficient length of time. The fact that many of them don't may be partly because of other life-style factors which give them protection, but is probably mainly a matter of pure luck. In the nutritional experiments on mice it is also true that all mice can be given cancer by exposing them to carcinogens, but that underfeeding can be powerfully protective.

Fitness foils cancer?

As I have mentioned, although the mice who were underfed were given only half as much calorie-containing food, or even less in some of the experiments, compared with the freely fed comparison group of mice, they remained in good health. A side-effect, however, seemed to be that in some instances they were subfertile. This is perhaps equivalent to the 'ballet dancer syndrome' in humans, the effect well known among athletes and dancers of lowered fertility (woman fail to have menstrual periods, for example) as a result of undereating and overexercising. It is fascinating to follow the comparison of the mice and humans a little further. As Dr Tannenbaum reported, the mice were sleek and active. They looked healthy and they lived longer. Possibly one reason for their slimness and activity was that they used up a great deal of energy searching in vain for food because they felt constantly hungry (though the lack of food did absolutely no harm to their health). It is inevitable that comparisons be made with the situation in humans: does over-feeding give us cancer too? In modern times in the affluent industrialised countries we can satisfy our appetites at any time of the day or night. Many of us are now in the position of the comparison group of Tannenbaum's mice, who were given unlimited access to food, and in whom much greater numbers of cancers developed.

Could it be possible then that physical activity helps prevent cancer? Certainly from the available evidence it would seem reasonable to suggest that people who cut down on calories, particularly in the form of fats, are likely to run a lower risk of getting cancer, and that those who also indulge in regular vigorous exercise may well protect themselves even further against certain forms of cancer.

The evidence on diet and cancer is still not considered hard and fast fact, and yet if you were to ask almost any person in possession of the basic information outlined here which of two people were more likely to get cancer: a fat person who takes little exercise, ets a great deal and whose diet is rich in fatty foods and low in dietary fibre, and a marathon runner who eats a modest wholefood diet, then most people would judge the latter 'sleeker' human to be at the lowest risk. This would in any case be the intuitive conclusion which many people might draw and, judging from the scientific evidence, incomplete though it is, this intuitive conclusion is surely the right one.

This is not to suggest that everybody should be encouraged to make drastic changes in their eating habits and lifestyle specifically in order to avoid cancer and possibly live 10 or 20 years longer. Smokers are often among the first to point out that a short but joyful life is preferable to a long and boring one! But there are others who want to develop at least some kind of awareness of the everyday health risks we run, whether from cancer, heart disease or any other potential cause of premature death. Until recent years we have been encouraged (partly because we have so much faith in the medical profession) to regard our bodies as the equivalent of motor cars, which need repairing when they break down, but which in other respects can be left alone. New thinking and new evidence on disease prevention now suggests that a large proportion of our health prospects and, perhaps even more significantly, those of our children, lie in our own hands.

Start now!

One of the fascinating findings reported by Tannenbaum was that underfeeding mice *after* the application of a carcinogen helped reduce the tumour-forming action of the treatment. This suggests that it is never too late to start restricting your diet! For if the same were found to apply to humans, then even when people have already been exposed to something which causes cancer, it is possible that a reduction in food, and in calories in particular, could prevent cancer from developing. This is pure guesswork at this stage, of course, but not wild by any means. Some tentative evidence is already available from cancer statistics from the Second World War period which suggest that frugal eating provided protection against the disease. Dr David Ingram at the University Medical Centre in Nedlands, Western Australia, recently studied the breast cancer statistics of England and Wales between the dates of 1928 and 1977. He found that at the onset of World War II there was a small reduction in breast cancer mortality at a time when people were eating far less sugar, meat and dairy products, and more cereals and vegetables, and he is not the first to suggest that the more frugal diet which rationing enforced might have had health benefits.

You will doubtless be relieved to find out that semi-starvation is not necessary in order to lower your cancer risks! Very recent experiments by Dr Mary Tucker of the Imperial Chemical Industries Laboratories at Alderley Park in Cheshire have shown that calorie restriction by only 20% (as opposed to around 50% in Tannenbaum's experiments) in rats and mice reduces the numbers of cancer tumours to less than half those experienced by animals allowed unlimited feeding of the same type of food. Although the reduction of calorie-containing food was only quite small, the effect on the development of cancer tumours was quite large (though not as large as in the Tannenbaum studies). Dr Tucker's research seems to show that, in mice at any rate, even cutting down quite modestly on food can have a large benefit. On a practical point, there is no doubt that the easiest way to cut down on total calorie intake is to reduce the kinds of foods which are the most concentrated sources of calories, namely sugary and fatty foods. If you then compensate by eating larger portions of foods in their natural form, such as wholemeal bread and fresh fruits or vegetables, you will almost certainly consume fewer total calories without even feeling you are on a diet! You will also gain whatever benefit extra fibre and vitamins provide. Dr Kenneth Heaton of Bristol University, England, has discovered that when people eat sweet foods and take drinks sweetened with sugar they consume about 25% more calories than people who eat other forms of carbohydrate. Since a standard-sized can of soft drink contains the equivalent of 10 lumps of sugar, if you wash down your meal with cola you may unwittingly take far more calories than you intended. But what is encouraging is that, *if* the experiments with mice can be compared with the human situation, just a small change – such as drinking natural fruit juice rather than manufactured drinks and eating more fruit in place of desserts high in fat and sugar – could make a big difference to your cancer risks.

5   Alcohol and additives, vitamins and vegetables

Alcohol has long been suspected as a cause of cancer, but the evidence for this is both enigmatic and intriguing. For one thing it seems almost certain that alcohol acting alone is not directly carcinogenic; only in combination with other circumstances is it definitely implicated as a specific cancer-causing agent. One of the most significant of these 'other circumstances' is smoking, since alcohol seems greatly to increase the risks of mouth, throat and gullet cancers among smokers over and above the extra risk they would already face from smoking alone.

Alcohol and cancer – a confirmed link

An obvious starting point when looking at alcohol as a possible cause of cancer is to study alcoholics. In France Drs Piquet and Tison reported as long ago as 1937 that among their patients with gullet cancer 19 out of every 20 were alcoholics, and since that time there has been plenty of confirmation about the role alcohol plays in causing this disease. The World Health Organisation concluded in 1964 that drinking alcohol was a *definitely established* cause of mouth, throat and gullet cancers. It is significant that it is named as a 'definite' culprit for which absolute proof of its role in causing cancer in conjunction with other factors – particularly tobacco – has been obtained. This makes it an agent about which we can now give firm advice as far as avoiding cancer is concerned. In their review of *The Causes of Cancer* in 1981, Doll and Peto endorsed the WHO finding and gave alcohol the dubious distinction of being a confirmed cancer cause accounting (they estimate) for three cases of fatal cancer out of every 100. This is far fewer than are strongly suspected to be caused by food, but the point is that the evidence against alcohol is precise enough for the case to be considered proven.

Which drinks are dangerous?

The evidence incriminating alcohol comes from a wide range of studies, and any brief account cannot do justice to all of them. The studies mostly consist of conducting surveys asking people about their drinking and looking simultaneously at the frequency of various types of cancers found among the people surveyed. Some of these investigations are undertaken among cancer patients, and a similar group of people not suffering from cancer are questioned as a comparison group. Other investigations look at entire communities in which very large surveys of people's drinking habits are carried out. This is completed either by questionnaires or by looking at the pattern of sales of different alcoholic drinks.

In Japan, for example, Drs Kono and Ikeda in 1979 looked at the amounts of various alcoholic drinks consumed in different parts of the country, and compared their findings with the causes of death among men in the same regions. They found an apparent relationship between the drinking of whisky and a strong Japanese drink called shochu and cancer of the gullet. Cancer of the rectum (the lowest part of the large bowel) seemed to be related to wine drinking, and cancer of the prostate also to shochu. Evidence of this sort cannot be taken as definite proof of carcinogenicity in itself, of course, because there may be relationships between the drinking of alcohol and other factors (for example, being wealthy enough to drink heavily may mean the person also eats a luxurious diet with plenty of rich foods), and these can confuse the issue. But this does not undermine the associations turned up by such surveys, especially if a sufficient number of surveys in different places all point more or less in the same direction. This has happened in the case of alcohol.

There is some disagreement about whether it is ethyl alcohol itself (the intoxicating component of alcoholic drinks) which causes cancer, or whether it is the presence of other substances in particular drinks which are carcinogenic. The balance of views seems to be that the over-riding effect of alcohol in helping to cause cancer does come from the action of ethyl alcohol, particularly when applied in conjunction with other substances such as tobacco smoke. But there are some important cases where other ingredients or impurities in particular types of alcoholic drink seem to be significant contributory causes. One such example occurs in Africa, a continent which yields some dramatic illustrations of how cancer incidence can vary from place to place, even over quite short distances, in a way which reflects the local drinking habits. The Oxford scientist Paula Cook discovered, for instance, that the drinking of African beer, brewed from maize, is strongly related to the incidence of cancer of the gullet. In western Kenya a great deal of African beer is drunk and this country has a very high incidence of this cancer, but in Uganda and Tanzania, where the maize 'home-brew' is not so popular, it is quite rare. An impurity of some sort in the maize beer is thought to be crucial to causing cancer, but the precise culprit has not yet been named.

France provides another classic example of a type of alcoholic drink in which a particular ingredient is thought to cause cancer. Dr Albert Tuyns of the International Agency for Research on Cancer in Lyon discovered in 1979 that a high incidence of cancer of the gullet existed in parts of Normandy among people who drank home-distilled apple brandy. It is, after all, remarkable that this type of cancer is much more common in France than in England, just a few kilometres across the Channel. Also in France a relationship between gullet cancer and the drinking of absinthe by alcoholics was reported as long ago as 1910 by Dr Lamy, and in China records for 1937 show that gullet cancer was then extremely common, accounting for half of all cancer cases. At that time a strong alcoholic drink known as pai-kan was generally held to be the cause. So individual associations between cancer and particular alcoholic drinks have been a feature of medical history for some time.

More recently the studies of Hinds and Kolonel in Hawaii in 1980 among five different ethnic groups have shown that beer drinking in particular is associated with a whole range of cancers, but in other places this association has not been corroborated. It seems likely that in this case pure alcohol itself is not a direct carcinogen, but that impurities in some types of beer are the real culprits. For example, it was discovered that beers in the United States contained nitroso compounds (see p. 87), which are known to be carcinogenic, and so the American government passed regulations to limit the amounts of these substances in beer. So some of the variation in different parts of the world concerning cancer and beer drinking may simply be the result of different amounts of such potentially carcinogenic contaminants. The nitroso compounds, for example, are among the culprits suspected as being the reason why people who drink African maize beer get more gullet cancer.

Any alcohol carries a risk

All this fascinating evidence about particular drinks being suspected causes of different cancers should not divert attention from the stronger evidence that *any form* of alcohol taken in large amounts carries a risk of causing cancer, particularly if you are a smoker. Apart from the evidence provided by alcoholics, a study by Dr Schwartz and his colleagues in France in the 1960s found that the more alcohol people drank (or admitted to drinking), the greater their chances of getting cancers of the mouth, throat and upper airways. It is not at all clear how alcohol acts in causing cancer, but it seems that the places which first come into contact with it, i.e. the mouth, throat and gullet, are most at risk. It is possible that alcohol alters the surface tissues in these parts of the body in a way which makes them more *susceptible* to developing cancer. The disease might in fact be triggered by other causes, such as food, tobacco smoke and contaminents in food and drink. A large majority of the cancer victims in Dr Schwartz's studies turned out to be heavy drinkers, and the same was reported from Finland in 1974 by Dr Hakulinen and his colleagues. They found that chronic male alcoholics suffered from more cases of cancers of the throat, gullet and lung than other Finnish men. It is very likely that the extra cases of lung cancer were caused by the extra number of cigarettes smoked by alcoholics – nearly always among the heaviest smokers. In the United States more than a dozen detailed surveys of cancer patients have been carried out, in which questions were asked about their alcohol intake and comparisons made with other groups of people, similarly questioned, who were not suffering from cancer but who were very similar in other respects to the cancer patients. These studies range from those of Dr Ernst Wynder in the 1950s right up to the 1970s and 1980s. The evidence collectively establishes a proven link between drinking large amounts of alcohol and being at risk of contracting cancers of the mouth, throat and gullet.

The role of alcohol in causing cancer is important for scientific reasons because it shows very clearly how two agents acting together can *multiply* the chances of causing cancer. The cancer-causing effect of tobacco in the mouth, throat and gullet is not merely *added* to the effect of alcohol on those parts of the body but *multiplied*, so that the effect of both drinking and smoking is many times greater than either indulgence alone (*see Fig 5*). It is perhaps unfortunate that most heavy drinkers also smoke, and that most smokers tend to smoke more cigarettes when they are drinking alcohol, so a strong warning about the significant hazard of drinking and smoking is appropriate.

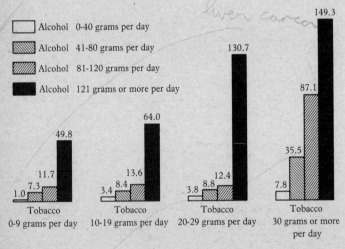

Fig 5 The risk of developing gullet cancer for a non-drinking non-smoker is defined as 1·0. As you can see from this chart, this means that a really heavy-drinking heavy smoker is well over 100 times more likely to develop this type of cancer than his abstemious counterpart. (Ten grams of alcohol are approximately equivalent to half a pint of beer *or* a single whisky *or* a small glass of wine. One cigarette contains about one gram of tobacco.)
(Redrawn from a paper by A. J. Tuyns *et al.* in the journal *Bull. Cancer (Paris)* Vol. 64 (1977).)

In 1979 Dr David Shottenfield of the Memorial Sloane Kettering Cancer Center in New York reported that drinking as little as two glasses of wine a day or just over a pint of beer (45 millilitres of alcohol) can increase the effect of tobacco in causing cancer. Until this report was published nobody had imagined that these hazardous activities when taken *in moderation* involved a high risk. Sir Richard Doll explains that the problem with advising people about the dangers of drinking alcohol is that there is no clear concept of how much is *too much*. Most people, he says, think that *too much* means: 'A little more than *I* drink'. My own conclusion is that, although there is some evidence that very small amounts of alcohol are good for helping prevent heart disease, it is impossible in practical terms to advise people how much is safe where cancer is concerned. The evidence tends to show that when alcohol is cheap, people drink more, so that a simple way of limiting alcohol consumption might be for the government to raise the level of taxation on it.

Liver cancer and alcohol

Alcohol is suspected as being one of the factors which can help cause liver cancer. By far and away the strongest evidence for this comes from the work of Dr Palmer Beasley in Taiwan, reported in the 1980s, which principally underlined the over-riding influence of hepatitis B infection in causing liver cancer in most victims, but which also identified alcohol as a contributory cause. The connection between alcohol and liver cancer has actually been suspected for a long time because alcohol causes cirrhosis, and this is thought often to be a necessary 'first stage' of illness which can then progress to liver cancer. Dr MacDonald at the Boston City Hospital, USA, reported in 1956 the relationship between the incidence of cirrhosis and that of liver cancer, and deduced that since cirrhosis in America was largely caused by alcohol, alcohol and liver cancer must also be linked. But just as tobacco and alcohol play a joint role in causing gullet cancer (alcohol on its own being unable to cause the disease, according to the statistics at least), it also seems likely that alcohol is not a direct carcinogen in the case of liver cancer either. It is more likely that it only causes cancer when something else is also influencing the liver. (One such likely agent is the mould-poison called aflatoxin, which I shall say more about later.) So it is not a simple statement of cause and effect: we cannot say directly that alcohol causes liver cancer, indeed most cases of the disease are probably predominantly caused by infection. But as a contributing cause, alcohol is high on the list of suspicious agents.

The indirect dangers of drinking

Another important indirect way in which alcohol is almost certainly deeply involved with causing cancer is through its effect on nutrition and eating behaviour. On the one hand there is the suggestion that for the majority of drinkers the effect of alcohol is likely to encourage over-eating which can lead to cancer, and on the other hand there is some evidence that heavy drinkers become severely malnourished and are more susceptible to cancer for that reason. Dr Paula Cook found in investigations in Iran that gullet cancer is strongly related to eating a diet containing very little in the way of fresh fruit and vegetables. Although alcohol is not the cause of such malnutrition in Iran, the same effect could in theory be produced among alcoholics who eat very little of anything, deriving most of their calories from alcohol. It is quite possible to use alcohol as your main energy source, because two glasses of wine a day provide 250 calories of energy. Several bottles of wine a day would give the alcoholic enough carbohydrate to satisfy his entire bodily requirements for energy.

But leaving aside the heavy drinkers, it is worth remembering that even moderate drinking adds calories to the diet, and if we drink every day as well as eating three square meals we run the risk of consuming too much carbohydrate. Alcohol is produced by fermentation from sugar, and there is not much difference between the calorie content of alcohol and the same weight of sugar. So all of the reservations voiced by pioneers such as Surgeon Captain Cleave about overconsumption and eating too much sugar (or white flour) in particular (which I explained in the last chapter) can be assumed to apply to alcohol just as much as to the sugar in your coffee or the delicious gâteau which rounds off your dinner.

Alcohol is also, like sugar, an easily absorbed carbohydrate. It has none of the reportedly beneficial dietary fibre content of other carbohydrate sources in more natural forms, such as wholemeal bread or potatoes. So alcohol emerges as a zero-fibre consumable, rich in calories, which leads to overeating, obesity and the whole range of cancers which have been linked to the 'overconsumption syndrome'. Not only does the drinker consume more calories, but he (or she) is far less likely to 'burn-off' these extra energy-giving calories by taking exercise. Heavy drinkers, and even moderate drinkers, know very well that exercise is more irksome the day after an evening's drinking. The drinker is more likely to sleep poorly and wake up late with less energy for the day's activities than his abstemious counterpart, so he is less likely to gain any protective effect conferred by exercise against cancer or any other disease. Drinking is indeed part of an unhealthy life-style, often featuring smoking, which is likely to lead in many indirect ways to a variety of cancers as well as the ones known to be produced in the parts of the body directly exposed to the alcohol.

Aflatoxin – the mould poison

The possibility that impurities or contaminants in alcoholic drinks may be involved in causing cancer suggests that it would be worth considering whether similar traces of impurities in food might also be a long-term cancer hazard. Although we in the West live at a time when controls have never been more rigorously applied to make sure our food is in the best possible condition and free from things which could make us ill, the type of impurity which causes cancer may not be excluded by such safeguards. This is because cancer hazards, as I have emphasised already, are mainly substances or circumstances to which we are exposed on a regular or even a continuous basis for a very long time. They may have no obvious short-term effect on human health, so that the most stringent industrial testing may not be able to show that they could cause cancer in the long term.

In the industrialised countries no obvious cancer hazards of this type have been identified yet, but we should not be complacent, and it is important for health organisations and governments to remain watchful. In the developing countries there is one particular food impurity which was recently shown to be a possible cause of liver cancer – the mould poison, aflatoxin. As I have mentioned, this is one of the leading candidates (along with hepatitis infection and alcohol) suspected of causing the very high incidence of liver cancer in hot, tropical countries. Aflatoxin is both a short- and a long-term poison produced by the mould *Aspergillus* which commonly affects stored foods such as groundnuts (peanuts) in places like West Africa. Because of its short-term poisonous action it first came to the attention of scientists in England when there was an outbreak of aflatoxin poisoning among turkeys who had eaten mouldy peanuts. This led to an intensive investigation of the effects of aflatoxin on animals, including checks on its cancer-causing ability. It did turn out to be carcinogenic in animals and since the mid 1960s (when this research began to be carried out) there has been concern that aflatoxin exposure could be a cancer risk for humans too. Mozambique has one of the highest liver cancer rates in the world, and it is perhaps not a co-incidence that people there have to eat stored foods, such as maize, for long periods of the year rather than fresh foods. During the 1983 drought in southern Africa, fears were expressed in the medical press that countries such as Zimbabwe – next door neighbour to Mozambique – may eventually suffer from an epidemic of liver cancer as a result of increasing numbers of people having to eat stored, rather than fresh grain which inevitably becomes contaminated with the *Aspergillus* mould. Although most people throw away the mouldy part of the food, aflatoxin traces can penetrate into the parts of the stored crop which are not obviously mouldy, so the only safeguard would be to refrain from eating any of it. This is obviously impossible in some circumstances, and it is clear that some cases of cancer may therefore result because people have had to choose between eating mouldy food, with its long-term risk of getting cancer, or, in the short term, dying of starvation.

In the richer countries it is also possible that some harm could come from eating food which has become partly mouldy. This is only a suspicion at this stage, but judging from the experience of the Third World it would seem prudent not to allow food to go mouldy and then simply cut away the mould. We cannot assume that traces of contamination in our foods are innocent until it has been proved so.

Bracken fern

Aflatoxin is an example of an impurity in food which causes cancer, but it is also possible that some of the normal trace constituents of certain foods may turn out to be a long-term cancer hazard. In Japan bracken fern is eaten as a delicacy and has been found to be associated with some cases of gullet cancer. The case against bracken fern is not fully proven, but it is interesting that in Argyll, West Scotland, Professor William Jarrett of Glasgow found in the 1970s that cows grazing on Scottish bracken suffered more frequently than other cows from digestive tract cancers. So far, however, there is no good evidence that bracken in the British countryside is any hazard to humans, but worries that cows might pass on the carcinogenic factor (whatever this is) in their milk have been expressed.

Nitroso compounds – leading cancer candidates

But what about traces of substances which are mixed with foods deliberately? Chemicals known as nitrates are widely used in farming as fertilisers, and both nitrates and similar chemicals called nitrites are used to help preserve food. Obviously these are very important for supplying us with enough food at the lowest possible price, and for making sure that bacteria and other dangerous micro-organisms do not infect the food once it has been prepared for us to buy and eat. As a result, we eat nitrates and nitrites in vegetables, fish and meats – especially cured meats, such as bacon. Unfortunately it has been discovered that the human gut is capable under some circumstances of converting nitrates and nitrites to the family of cancer-causing agents known as N-nitroso compounds.

Governments have been aware for some years that the preservatives and farm chemicals containing nitrates and nitrites are a potential hazard and in the United States the Committee on Nitrite and Alternative Curing Agents in Food reported to the National Academy of Sciences in 1981 on the possible harm such food additives might be causing. The average amounts of nitrate and nitrite consumed in different foods were estimated, and the reassuring conclusion given that up until now there has been no indication that these are causing significant increases in cancer rates. The subject is complicated by the fact that many foods, such as vegetables, also naturally contain substances which can strongly affect the formation of nitroso compounds. Vitamin C, for example, is known to inhibit this process and might therefore protect against any cancer hazard that added nitrates possibly present.

Although there is not much evidence that N-nitroso compounds from food in places such as America are significantly involved in causing cancer, these substances are strongly under suspicion in other parts f the world. In the Transkei region of South Africa, for example, the presence of nitrosamine in African beer has been put forward as a possible explanation for a particularly high rate of cancer of the gullet (though there has been no proof of this). It is therefore not possible to give complete reassurance that preservatives and N-nitroso compounds which can be formed from them are free from any cancer hazard. It may well be better, however, to accept a small amount of contamination by preservatives in the interests of keeping vegetables in good condition since most surveys seem to show that vegetables help protect against cancer and therefore, even if preserved, probably do more good than harm. It would be quite wrong to cut down on your intake of vegetables because they are the principle source of nitrates, which have by no means been definitely proved to cause cancer. A better way to reduce your intake of such preservatives would be to cut down on smoked and cured meats and fish: this would also help reduce fat intake which is a sound recommendation for avoiding cancer.

Additives

As well as preservatives, we are familiar with a wide range of other food additives: thickeners, flavour enhancers, emulsifiers, colourings, to name a few, and we are less familiar with a whole range of yet more permitted additives: acidulants, leavening agents, stabilisers, anti-oxidants and many others. Modern food technology is based upon the aim (among others) of making the foods which are easily available into products which people will want to buy, and doing so at a price which people can afford. It is no good having a foodstuff which is extremely healthy and free from all risks of causing cancer or any other disease if nobody finds it enjoyable to eat. But the substances which are added to create the food products with which we are familiar have often come under scrutiny as possible causes of cancer. The American National Research Council's report on *Diet, Nutrition and Cancer* (1982) points out that there are nearly 3000 substances intentionally added to 'process foods' in the USA, and another 12 000 chemicals, such as those used in food packaging, are classified as 'indirect additives'. Only a very small proportion of these have ever been thoroughly tested on a long-term basis for their potential ability to cause cancer. The report actually concludes that there is 'no evidence that the increasing use of food additives has contributed significantly to the overall risk of cancer for humans', but the scientists do issue a warning: because the additives have only been used in comparatively recent times, we cannot yet be sure that they are completely free from cancer-causing effects.

Perhaps the most universal food additive is sugar. Even 'savoury' foods like tomato ketchup contain a very large proportion of sugar, as do many of the other sauces and 'relishes' used at the table. Sugar also finds its way into a wide range of canned and preserved foods – sweet or savoury – as a glance at the ingredients list will show. So this additive is consumed in very large quantities, in addition to the amount many people take in their tea or coffee and in obviously sweet things like sweets, biscuits and desserts. Sugar is such an accepted additive, an 'old friend', that we don't expect it to be a danger, but it contributes to 'overconsumption' and the excessive intake of calories (discussed in the last chapter) which are themselves thought to be significant 'risk factors' for cancer. The market forces which have shaped our food industry have encouraged manufacturers to add sugar to almost everything, so if you want to avoid this additive you will have to read the small print very carefully or stick to foods which are not highly processed.

Another universal and familiar food additive is salt. There is no doubt that since processed foods have become available the average intake of salt in industrialised countries has increased greatly. Professor J. V. Joosens of the School of Public Health in Leuven, Belgium, has looked into the relationship between the amount of salt eaten in various places and the incidence of stomach cancer and has made out a case for suggesting that salt is involved in causing this disease. Even though there has not been much corroborating evidence for this, it is certainly true that we do not *need* to eat the amounts of salt which are typical of the average person's diet today, and as it is also thought to be involved in causing strokes and other circulatory illnesses, there are reasonable grounds for suggesting that a reduction of salt as part of the 'prudent diet' is advisable. (Indeed this is already being suggested in the United States and, in Britain, by the Royal College of Physicians, as one of the ways in which we might hope to avoid heart and circulatory diseases.)

The promise of vitamins

As I explained in Chapter 4, one of the reasons for the current wave of enthusiasm for dietary fibre is that there seems to be a possibility that it can give protection against certain types of cancer, just as it certainly does give protection against a range of other diseases, particularly those affecting the large bowel. The hope is that fibre is something which people can add to their diets without having to worry about reducing other types of food. This is obviously an advantage if you are trying to persuade people to change their eating habits: it is always easier to add something new rather than to try to persuade people to give up something they enjoy. It now seems there is another class of substances present in food which could easily be increased if they could be proved to help protect against cancer – namely, the vitamins.

Vitamins are not foods in themselves, being required only in minute quantities by the body, but they make it possible for certain chemical reactions to take place inside us without which we would die. Up until the 1950s and even the 1960s the majority view among nutritionists was that vitamins are probably required only in quantities large enough to avoid the well known vitamin-deficiency diseases such as scurvy (lack of vitamin C), rickets (lack of vitamin D), and so on. But there have been dissenting voices. Professor Linus Pauling in Stanford, California (holder of two Nobel prizes), has for many years held the view that the ideal intake of vitamins needed to maintain the best possible health has never been properly investigated. He points out that community health experts have always been concerned with the short-term (and very drastic) ill effects observed among people who don't consume even the minimum amount needed of certain vitamins. He believes that in fact much larger amounts may eventually be proved to be of extreme benefit to our health, perhaps even making it possible to live a decade or more longer than at present.

In the case of vitamin A there is a problem involved in increasing your intake: it is moderately poisonous. Too much vitamin D can also cause illness, so obviously the idea of increasing the amount of any vitamin in your diet has to be viewed with caution. Vitamin C seems to be quite safe, however, even in very much larger doses than is recommended for warding off scurvy. To avoid scurvy humans need about 25 milligrams of vitamin C every day; but (as is often recommended for the treatment of the common cold) the dose can be increased tenfold or even a hundredfold without any ill effects.

Both vitamin C and vitamin A (retinol), and other compounds which are converted into vitamin A in the body after being eaten (such as carotene), are thought to be capable of preventing cancer. Other vitamins, too, have been investigated in humans and tested in animals for their potential ability to ward off this disease. In all cases, the hope is that a benefit could exist in adding these substances to our diet which would then make it less important for people to change long-held eating habits in other ways in the interests of preventing cancer.

Vitamins and vegetables

So what is the evidence about vitamins and cancer? The most powerful evidence comes from research based on surveying the food different groups of people eat and comparing their cancer rates. There is almost no evidence at all at present that taking vitamin pills alone can prevent the disease, and this is a question which hopefully will be finally resolved by more dedicated research involving animal studies and human surveys in the future. What we do know is that the types of food which contain vitamin A and the types of food which contain vitamin C are eaten more often by people who tend to get less cancer. This does not at this stage prove that either vitamin A or vitamin C has any protective effect, because it could be some other substance in these foods which matters, but the whole field of study looks fascinating. Milk and liver contain vitamin A, and a whole range of vegetables contain compounds such as carotene (including carrots, as you might deduce from the name of this substance) which can be converted in the body into vitamin A. It is worth noting at this point that green leafy vegetables such as cabbage also contain chemicals called 'indoles' which are considered to be possibly active in preventing cancer. All we are really sure of at the moment is that people who eat a lot of vegetables get less cancer.

In 1975 Dr Erik Bjelke reported his finding that among a large group of men he had questioned about eating habits, lung cancer was less common in those who ate vegetables containing vitamin A sources. This was even true for smokers, so green leafy vegetables seem to be a way of helping smokers to avoid lung cancer – good news indeed for those who have not been able to quit. Since Dr Bjelke's findings there has been a flurry of interest in the protective effect of eating vegetables against a variety of cancers. The idea that green leafy vegetables protect against lung cancer was further confirmed in Singapore by Dr MacLennan in 1977 who found that a particular group of Chinese women, known to be at high risk of getting lung cancer, seemed to be protected if they ate vegetables of the sort Erik Bjelke found to be protective, namely those which contain sources of vitamin A. A range of evidence from many other centres adds to the suggestion that vitamin A and carotene offer some protection not only against lung cancer but against cancers of the larynx, bladder, gullet, stomach and perhaps other types too.

One of the main problems with these studies is that the scientists can only gather the information that particular foods are eaten (and even then the accuracy depends on the memory of patients or volunteers in such surveys). The surveys do not prove conclusively that it is actually the vitamin A in these foods which provides the protection against cancer. A very interesting study in this area is the work of Paula Cook of Oxford, already mentioned, who in 1979 surveyed the diet of people living near the Caspian Sea in Iran. She investigated this region because of the exceptionally high incidence of cancer of the gullet suffered by communities there. It was suspected that food could be one of the main reasons for this type of cancer being so common, and the survey showed that the people most affected were those who ate the least fresh fruit and fresh, green, leafy vegetables, and were therefore deficient in vitamins A and C. But these foods contain many other nutrients and trace elements, any of which might prove to be helpful in preventing cancer. Vitamins A and C seem to be the most likely candidates, but it would be better (on present knowledge) to recommend eating the foods themselves, rather than vitamin tablets.

The possibility that vitamin A may also protect against stomach cancer was implied by the work of Dr Takeshi Hirayama in Japan, the country with the highest incidence of stomach cancer in the world. He made a study of a quarter of a million healthy people and monitored them, noting any who developed cancer. His results showed that people who drink milk every day (a source of vitamin A) are less likely to suffer from stomach cancer, and that non-smokers who eat green and yellow vegetables develop stomach cancer less commonly than people who do not eat these foods regularly.

How vitamin A is thought to prevent cancer

One of the reasons that scientists are so excited about vitamin A and the possibility that it can prevent cancer is that this substance is normally involved in the process of renewal within the body, in which living cells reproduce themselves to replace layers of tissue which are worn out. The skin and the lining of the gut are both examples of parts of the body where continual renewal of the surface layers is going on. When we eat, part of the gut lining gets carried away with the food during digestion and passes out with the stools. A new surface layer is continually being manufactured by means of automatic reproduction of the living cells making up this tissue. Skin, too, is continually being renewed to provide us with an effective covering which isolates the inner tissues of our bodies from our harmful and germ-laden environment. When there is not enough vitamin A present in the body the tissues regenerate in an abnormal way, forming a pattern of differently textured cells described as 'metaplasia'. It is also known that metaplasia often precedes cancer. Indeed one of the most effective methods for the early detection of cancer of, for example, the cervix is to look for a form of metaplasia. It has been known from animal experiments since the 1960s that vitamin A supplements can prevent metaplasia from occurring after a cancer-causing agent has been administered, and experiments with aflatoxin also show that vitamin A can stop some of the cancer-causing effects of this mould poison. These facts are a great spur to investigators who believe that the amount of vitamin A we eat could make a difference to whether we do or do not get the disease.

Synthetic vitamin A

Because vitamin A is poisonous to humans in large quantities there is a lot of interest among pharmaceutical companies in the idea of synthesising a compound which is equivalent to it but which is not poisonous. A wide range of vitamin A-like compounds, called retinoids, have been manufactured and in animals they do seem to exert an anti-cancer effect similar to that of natural vitamin A (retinol). But although these developments are interesting I suggest that the idea of reaching for the pill bottle as a means of preventing cancer is a little naïve. Cancer has complex causes, with often more than one factor acting in concert to cause the development of a tumour. The only firm evidence from human studies that we have is that eating certain foods is associated with getting less cancer, and it may well be that the benefit is as much concerned with other constituents of these foods (if not more so) as with their ability to supply the body with vitamin A. There are other confusing issues about the evidence concerning diet. People who eat a lot of vegetables may well eat less meat, cheese and dairy produce because they don't need to satisfy their appetites on such foods, being satiated with vegetables. This automatically means they have less fat in their diet, which probably helps protect against some of the common cancers irrespective of whether the vegetables give any extra protective effect.

The best way to make practical use of the available information about diet and cancer is to form judgements, albeit on the basis of incomplete evidence, about the broad balance of your diet, rather than trying to be absolutely certain that nothing you eat can give you cancer. In fact there is every reason to believe that you can eat almost anything on an occasional basis and not risk getting cancer (even bracken fern, for example). The problem only really arises when you *continually* consume foods which on the balance of the available evidence seem to be implicated as long-term cancer hazards.

Vegetables are good for you

On this basis there is a lot to be said for eating more green leafy vegetables such as spinach, cabbage, lettuce, broccoli and other members of this group (*Brassica*), and also yellow and orange vegetables, such as carrots, peppers and pumpkin. I find it interesting that American food, for example, is usually accompanied by good fresh salads and plenty of succulent fresh fruits. Although it is still the fourth most common cause of cancer death, today's stomach cancer rate in America is only a fraction of what it was earlier in the century when more Americans died from stomach cancer than any other form of the disease. I can't help drawing the conclusion that the wider availability of fresh fruits and salads is involved in this, especially since a good deal of statistical evidence from dietary surveys suggests that eating these foods helps protect against stomach cancer. Dr Meinsma in Holland, for instance, reported in 1964 that stomach cancer patients were less likely to have been in the habit of eating citrus fruits than similar people who did not suffer from cancer, and since that time a body of work from Dr William Heanszel and Dr Pelayo Correa in America, from Dr Erik Bjelke in Norway, and from Dr Lawrence Kolonel's studies of five ethnic groups in Hawaii have all endorsed the idea that the sorts of foods which contain vitamin C, such as fruits and raw vegetables, help protect against stomach cancer. There is also a convincing scientific explanation of why vitamin C itself may be responsible for this protection – it can prevent the formation in the stomach of the feared N-nitroso compounds from nitrates in the diet. Together with the findings of Paula Cooke in Iran about gullet cancer being less likely among people who get enough fresh fruit and vegetables, and the long-standing views of authoritative scientific 'elder statesmen' such as Dr Linus Pauling, a case could even be made out for encouraging people to take vitamin C pills. But the only *firm* recommendation for avoiding stomach and other cancers thought to be involved with vitamin C is by eating the foods which contain it, rather than hoping that the isolated vitamin will have the same protective effect.

The safest dietary recommendation at present is to eat the sorts of foods which contain vitamin C (fresh fruits and raw vegetables) and the sorts of food which contain vitamin A and carotene. The vegetable sources of carotene also contain vitamin C and many dietary surveys show that people who eat them are less likely to get cancer. But the animal sources of vitamin A (milk and liver, for example) should be taken only in moderation because such foods are also sources of fat which is not recommended in large amounts to anybody wanting to stay healthy.

The Interim Dietary Advice

Scientists who are trying to solve the many problems of understanding what precise aspects of diet are responsible for causing or preventing cancer are in a difficult position today. On the one hand they are convinced that food is one of the biggest causes of cancer in the world, and they have a lot of evidence which points the finger of suspicion at certain types and trace substances. Yet they seem to be frightened of making fools of themselves by recommending people to eat or avoid such foods, only to be proved wrong a few years later as more information is uncovered.

They also feel they have a responsibility for giving sound information rather than mere speculation, and this has all contributed to a great reluctance among them to publicise their findings widely. The field of study is also quite hard to understand. The point that the foods containing vitamins A and C may protect against cancer but that it is not necessarily the vitamins themselves which provide the protective action is a difficult concept to get across, and it is quite understandable that scientists prefer to retreat to their laboratories until the whole picture has become clearer and more definite. But in the meantime people all over the world are exposing themselves to foods which are *already prime suspects* for causing cancer. So what is to be done?

The committee of the US National Research Council's report on *Diet, Nutrition and Cancer* (1982) decided that despite the fact that the evidence is incomplete, it was time to make recommendations to the public. The scientists compiling the report formed balanced judgements about a number of aspects of our diet and gave their conclusions on both the state of knowledge about cancer-causing foods and the most effective ways of tackling the food/cancer problem. Clearly there is a need for the public to be told about the dietary avoidance of cancer, and the committee members drew a comparison with another scientific discipline: weather forecasting. In both cases the public demands information and the scientists are obliged to give it as accurately as possible, bearing in mind the uncertainties.

So here are the 'interim dietary guidelines' published by the committee, which should be regarded in a similar light to the 'interim weather forecast' made by meteorological scientists on the basis of incomplete but nevertheless exhaustively researched evidence. In other words you can be fairly certain that in broad terms the guidelines are correct, and any small details which turn out to be inaccurate as more information is accumulated over the years must be excused at this stage, for to withhold information now would be to deprive the public of facts which seem to be crucial to their long-term survival.

• First and foremost is the evidence that eating too much fat can cause breast and bowel cancer, and possibly other cancers too. It is well worth noting that the evidence that heart disease is also caused by eating too much fat is overwhelming. So reducing fats in the diet should be the first priority by, for example, choosing lean meats, low fat cheeses and vegetarian dishes – a subject I elaborate upon in the final chapter.

● Vegetables, fruits and wholegrain cereal foods are associated with reduction of the risk of many cancers and are firmly recommended by the American committee as a prudent choice for avoiding cancer.

● Less firmly, the scientists warn that salt-cured, salt-pickled and smoked foods may introduce compounds which can be converted into such carcinogens as the N-nitroso compounds in the gullet and stomach and thus should be eaten in moderation.

● The committee also warns against eating too much food which has been contaminated in any way, or which has been preserved by the use of chemicals which could be involved in causing cancer. This warning should be taken as a plea for moderation rather than abstinence, however, and, as I have already mentioned, you must weigh the benefits against the potential hazards and thus probably choose to eat vegetables and fruits even if the only ones available to you have been stored or preserved.

● Last, and by no means least, is a warning against drinking too much alcohol, particularly if you smoke. As the second biggest *definitely confirmed* cause of human cancer death this warning must be taken seriously, and since tobacco and alcohol are causes of a wide spectrum of other illnesses, there are good reasons for avoiding them quite apart from the desire to avoid cancer.

● Dietary fibre does not get a specific mention in the 'interim dietary guidelines' I have reviewed here, although it is implied to some extent in those on wholegrain cereals, fruits and vegetables. Because there is still a confusion between 'crude fibre' (which is the food residue which can accurately be measured by dissolving foods in acid and alkali) and 'dietary fibre' (which is the food residue which passes undigested into the large bowel), there is not yet full agreement in the international research information about the protective role of dietary fibre against bowel cancer. I am personally convinced by the research of Burkitt, Cleave and others that fibre is important, as are many other scientists, and I suggest that a diet rich in whole unprocessed foods in their natural state, as Cleave recommended, automatically fulfills most of the 'interim dietary guidelines' advanced here for avoiding cancer.

6 Women's cancers, hormones and the pill

There are inequalities between the sexes which in some respects make it difficult for women to avoid certain types of cancer. Some modern developments have actually increased the risks of certain cancers among women, and it could be argued that the 'fair sex' has been getting a raw deal, being persuaded to adopt life-styles which the evidence suggests are risky in health terms.

Women have fairly similar rates to men as far as cancers of the bowel and stomach are concerned and, now that women smoke, they run a very high risk of getting lung cancer, previously confined mainly to men. But there are other cancers where differences in incidence between the sexes are enormous. Breast cancer accounts for about a quarter of all cancer in British women, and both womb and ovarian cancers account for a significant minority of female cases. Breast cancer is very rare in men, however, and, of course, womb and ovarian cancer absent, so that these three gynaecological cancers (accounting for four out of every 10 cancers among women) are almost exclusively female afflictions. They probably each have different causes, and it is clear that women may need to adopt special strategies for avoiding them.

Breast cancer caused by Western life-style?

Although breast cancer is already common (and is becoming slightly more common) in Europe and North America, it is rare in places such as Africa and other areas of the Third World, and rare also in oriental countries, including Japan – an advanced industrialised society. Eating habits are therefore likely to be important causes of such differences, particularly the eating of foods rich in calories, whether from fats or from carbohydrates, especially refined carbohydrates such as white sugar and flour. But there are other reasons for the international differences in breast cancer statistics which are now better understood.

Pregnancy affects breast cancer risks

It is not surprising to medical scientists that being overweight carries a small extra risk of breast cancer, and that the disease is most common in countries where a great deal of fat-containing food is eaten. This is because body fat and fats in the intestine can be converted into the body chemicals (hormones) known as oestrogens which are related to female sexuality. It has been known for a long time that oestrogen is an important influencing factor in connection with female cancers. High blood levels of oestrogen can help cause forms of the disease (such as when the hormone is prescribed as a drug) and having a deficiency of oestrogen can help prevent them (such as when the ovaries, which produce this hormone, are removed in young women). But the picture is complicated. First pregnancy at an early age (during the teens and twenties) helps protect against breast cancer even though circulating levels of oestrogen during pregnancy are much higher than in a woman who is not pregnant. The risk of breast cancer is slightly increased by first pregnancy above the age of about 35, however, which suggests that in this older group of women oestrogen might be involved in helping to cause the disease. In a woman who does not get pregnant there is a regular monthly cycle of oestrogen levels (and other body chemicals) and it may well be the interruption of this cycle rather than the absolute levels of oestrogen in young women which improves cancer risks. This may sound confusing, but the important fact to bear in mind is that oestrogen seems to play a central role in the formation of cancer. It even helps many types of breast cancer tumours to develop (these grow more slowly when deprived of oestrogen). So it is highly important to focus attention upon oestrogen and to look for ways of manipulating this hormone in order to minimise the risks of cancer.

Let's take a look at some of the available evidence. For one thing it has been noticed that women who never have babies tend to be at a higher risk of getting breast cancer. (Reports about the frequency of breast cancer among nuns go back to the nineteenth century and before, when doctors already realised that the excess risk of the disease among such women was probably related to their celibacy.) This in turn is probably related to the concentrations of hormones (including oestrogen, already mentioned, and others such as prolactin) circulating in the blood at different times of life. These all-important levels of hormones in the female body are governed not only by pregnancy, but also by lactation and the use of various drugs – including the contraceptive pill.

Another area of risk is thought possibly to be related to the number of menstrual periods in a woman's lifetime. The early onset of periods (the menarche), i.e. before the age of, say, 12, is a known risk factor for breast cancer later in life. So too is a late 'change of life' (menopause). A combination of early menarche and late menopause increases the number of menstrual periods a women has in her life and this seems to be another risk factor for breast cancer. Pregnancy reduces the number of menstrual periods and so cuts down this risk. In addition, the mere condition of pregnancy (but not, apparently, of lactation) supplements the protective effect of missing nigh on a year's worth of periods, with early pregnancy giving the most extra protection.

At the extremes, if you take the average risk of breast cancer as being that facing a woman who has her first child in her late twenties, then a woman who had a child shortly after the onset of periods is only one third as likely to develop breast cancer later in life as the 'average' woman. Someone having her first baby after the age of 35 would experience a slightly increased risk (about an extra 30%) compared to the average woman. So the most likely person to get breast cancer is a woman whose periods began before the age of 12, who either never had a child or had a first pregnancy after the age of 35, and whose change of life occurred at an age of more than 50 years. To this can be added the fact that being overweight also increases the risk. On a more speculative basis, the use of 'hormone replacement therapy' (oestrogen therapy) during and after the menopause and, possibly, the contraceptive pill are also involved in the complex of factors which go together to increase the risk of breast cancer.

The so-called 'Western way of life' includes certain attitudes towards pregnancy (that it should be delayed, if possible, often well into the third decade of life) and family size (to be kept as small as possible in the interests of economy). These attitudes encourage behaviour which research suggests increases female breast cancer risks. It is therefore not surprising that the breast cancer rates are higher in such countries than in the Third World. A recent study confirmed the relationship in one Western country in particular – the United States – between these aspects of Western life and the pattern of breast cancer. Reported in 1980 by Dr William Blot, of the National Cancer Institute in Bethesda, Maryland, this study showed a clear rise in recent years in breast cancer rates affecting women after the change of life. This, he explains, appears to be related to 'changing patterns of childbearing among young adult women over the first two thirds of this century'. By this he was specifically referring to the tendency among women during this century to have babies at a later age than was popular during the last century, and so the report confirms the protective effect of an early first pregnancy. Previous work by Professor Brian MacMahon and others found that having a baby before the age of 18 makes a woman about one third as likely to develop breast cancer as a woman who has her first child at 35.

Blot's statistics were derived from an analysis of census information about women during the twentieth century from the whole of the United States of America, combined with information about deaths caused by breast cancer. He was therefore able to pinpoint 'societal customs concerning childbearing' as the single most important factor affecting breast cancer rates in the United States. He suggested that the recent fall in deaths from breast cancer in the United States is most likely to be the result of the post-World War II rise in pregnancies – the 'baby boom'.

Breast cancer is hormone-dependent

The part the hormone oestrogen plays in established (i.e. already diagnosed) breast cancer strongly supports the idea that it also helps to cause the disease in the first place. For one thing, in the treatment of breast cancer it has been discovered that removal of the ovaries (oophorectomy) causes a marked reduction in the rate of breast cancer growth. As the ovaries are the main source of oestrogen within the body, it seems clear that removing this source deprives the tumours of oestrogen upon which they appear to be dependent. This idea has been borne out in recent years by studies in which breast cancer patients were given a drug which has the opposite effect of oestrogen in the body – anti-oestrogen therapy – and this had a similar effect on some breast tumours, though not all. Breast cancer is widely described as a hormone-dependent disease. This is not to suggest that hormones are the only factor influencing its development, but oestrogen certainly does seem to be an important promoter of the growth of certain tumours.

The two forms of breast cancer

To understand the nature of breast cancer risks more clearly, it is important to know that there are two distinct categories of th disease: the rare pre-menopausal breast cancer, which can strike women even as young as in their twenties, and post-menopausal breast cancer, which accounts for by far the largest numbers of breast cancer cases. The 'protection' against breast cancer provided by having a baby during teenage is largely protection against the latter, more common form of the disease. (A wide body of evidence about other matters, such as diet, which affect the risk of breast cancer in late middle age, also seems to pinpoint the teenage years as being the most important period for influencing breast cancer risks.) Oestrogen probably affects both forms of breast cancer, although many facts have yet to be discovered about the precise pattern of this effect. Diet can influence hormone levels because the wrong one can make a person fat, which itself causes the body to produce more oestrogen. This is one reason why it is important for scientists to examine further the possibility that food eaten by children can influence breast cancer risks later in life.

The pill and breast cancer

One of the most worrying aspects of breast cancer risks is the possibility that early use of the contraceptive pill may turn out to be a factor. The clever idea behind the invention of the contraceptive pill was that the doses it contained of oestrogen and progesterone would simulate the natural effects of pregnancy. In the human body the effect of taking these compounds regularly is to suppress the natural bodily processes necessary for conception (just as they are suppressed during pregnancy) and to smooth out the monthly cycle of varying hormone levels. This seemed such an apparently safe form of contraception that the medical authorities, after wide-ranging tests on animals and humans, felt that the risk of there being any danger in the method was so small that it could be widely recommended. The situation has not changed dramatically since then, but birth control pills containing oestrogen and progesterone-like compounds are now so widely used all over the world that possible long-term hazards are constantly being looked into very carefully, especially since most forms of cancer take a long time to develop. In the case of the type of breast cancer which strikes later in life it seems that processes which take place in adolescence may contribute towards planting the seeds of this disease, and these do not germinate until several decades later, perhaps not until old age. The contraceptive pill could be just such a seed.

A report published in *The Lancet* in 1983 by Professor Malcolm Pike and his colleagues at the University of Southern California in Los Angeles announced that use of certain formulations of the pill (those having a high progestogen component) were associated with an increased risk of breast cancer. In this report it is stated that only women who took the pill before the age of 25 and for several years are at risk (five years of pill-taking gives a four-fold increased risk), and that pills having a low progestogen component – which includes most present formulations – do not appear to increase the risk of breast cancer.

The report provoked a storm of protest in medical circles, because other studies have tended to exonerate the pill as far as breast cancer risks are concerned. One reason for having confidence in the pill's safety is the fact that the daily dose of oestrogen suspends the natural menstrual cycle, just as happens in pregnancy, so it was thought that it would mirror the protective effect against breast cancer which pregnancy seems to give. (The breakthrough bleeding that occurs when a woman stops taking the pill for one week out of every four is not actually a normal period, but a 'signal' to reassure her she is not pregnant.) You might therefore expect using the pill from an early age to help protect against breast cancer later in life, just as does having a baby. But the results of Professor Pike's team certainly do not give any reassurance that this is so. Their initial findings suggest the opposite, in fact, and in the long term we simply do not know what the effects of using the pill from a very early age are likely to be. Medical scientists are already familiar with the fact that artificially produced chemicals which are designed to imitate natural body chemicals (such as hormones) certainly do not invariably possess *all* of the same effects as the natural compound. It would be remarkable if the oestrogen in contraceptive pills, which is a synthetic substance not extracted from humans, had *exactly* the same effects as natural oestrogen, and other components of the pill, such as progestogen, may be just as important as far as breast cancer risks are concerned. The pill has only been in use for about 20 years so there are not yet sufficient women old enough to be at risk of the commonest form of breast cancer, *post*-menopausal breast cancer, to show up any trend. It may turn out that the pill only has an effect on the far less common *pre*-menopausal breast cancer.

We shall not find out the answers to these worries for another 20 or 30 years, but the evidence so far suggests that it would be prudent to give a great deal more thought to the use of the birth control pill, especially for very young women. It is ironic that it is during a woman's teens and early twenties that taking the pill seems to be most risky since that is the time when she is most likely to want to use it. Young women of the 'pill generation' have been able for the first time to explore their sexuality without risk of pregnancy by using a form of contraception which is simple to use and extremely reliable. It will be hard for them to give it up. As a result of the scare which followed Professor Pike's report health officials are now worried that fears about the pill may lead to an increase in unwanted pregnancies, and this is the dilemma constantly facing doctors who are trying to do their best for patients. At present it simply cannot be predicted how much the early use of the pill increases the chances of breast cancer later in life, or even whether it does at all. The precise formulation of the pill may be crucial to this, and the advantages gained by the use of oral contraception have always to be borne in mind.

Hormone Replacement Therapy

Another medical dilemma faces doctors who are trying to advise patients about the need for 'hormone replacement therapy'. This involves giving women oestrogen-like drugs to replace the body's natural oestrogen after the menopause, and can make a dramatic difference to the lives of women who suffer 'hot flushes', depression and a whole range of other medical problems during this difficult time of life. (Not all women experience a difficult menopause, however. Some have few symptoms, if any.) Unfortunately studies have definitely shown that this treatment can help to cause the type of cancer which begins in the womb. As far as breast cancer is concerned the risk is not so clear, but several reports are beginning to suggest that long-term use of 'menopausal oestrogens' can add to the risk of contracting this disease too. However, in the serious medical condition called osteoporosis, which almost exclusively affects women, and which involves loss of bone mass resulting in brittleness of the bones and often multiple fractures of the spine, the use of oestrogens is a valid treatment and can halt the progress of the disease. Many women might wish to take the risk of cancer in order to avoid the extreme hardship of severe osteoporosis. Hormone replacement therapy also seems to reduce the risks of heart attack, so there are 'checks and balances'. In medicine, decisions are sometimes not clear cut, and no absolute rules can be given. But by understanding the precise risks of different treatments patients can at least make more informed decisions about their future. Certainly the wave of enthusiasm for this treatment (originally hailed as an elixir of youth) has declined, even in the United States where it has been most popular.

Radiation and breast cancer

There is no doubt that radiation can occasionally cause breast cancer. The atomic bombing of Hiroshima at the close of the Second World War caused increased rates of the disease even among those women who had received quite small doses (as little as 10 rads). This is no more than patients undergoing complicated tests used to receive in hospital in the past when given a long series of X-rays.

One recent study confirming earlier work which suggested that radiation is a cause of breast and other cancers was carried out by Dr Keith Baverstock of the Harwell Research Establishment near Oxford, England. He found that women who painted luminous instruments during World War II using paint containing substances which produce atomic radiation were more likely to develop breast cancer than women not exposed to this substance. A range of other investigations have come to much the same conclusion, with the finding that the most vulnerable period in a woman's life seems to be during adolescence and that there is a time lag of about 15 years between exposure to radiation and the diagnosis of breast cancer. Also, the simple fact has been established that the risk rises exactly with the amount of exposure: twice as much radiation gives double the risk of breast cancer, and there is no guarantee that even very small amounts of radiation do not involve a risk – there does not seem to be a threshold below which radiation exposure is safe.

Having said this it is important to point out that although radiation definitely causes breast and other cancers, the risk is very small even when the dose of radiation is quite large. This was shown clearly by the results of Professor Sir Richard Doll of the University of Oxford and Peter Smith of the London School of Hygiene and Tropical Medicine recently in the latest of a series of reports following up the incidence of cancer among people who were treated with radiation therapy for the arthritic condition known as ankylosing spondilitis earlier this century. Even though many thousands of patients were treated with quite large doses of radiation there were only a few cases of cancer, so your chances of avoiding cancer despite being exposed to radiation are very high. Nevertheless this is one more risk factor which adds to others present in your life-style, and the art of avoiding cancer is to keep these various risks in proper perspective and eliminate or reduce them all so far as is possible or convenient.

Breast screening

There has been a tremendous wave of enthusiasm in the United States recently for breast cancer screening: in other words regular X-ray examinations for healthy women to make sure they do not have any signs of breast cancer. There is also constant interest about methods of 'breast self-examination' by which women can find lumps or abnormalities in their breasts at the earliest possible stage. All this is based on the hope that if the disease is caught early enough treatment will be more successful. There are reasonable grounds for moderate optimism that catching the disease early may indeed help in curing it. But these grounds are not yet proven and it should be remembered that the X-ray examinations used to screen for breast cancer (mammography) could also occasionally cause the disease.

The main reasons for hope about screening at present come from a study of women screened for breast cancer undertaken by an American insurance company, the Health Insurance Plan. One of the latest assessments of the success of the HIP study appears in the *Journal of the National Cancer Institute*, and was written by Dr Sam Shapiro of the Johns Hopkins University in Baltimore, Maryland. The importance of the study is that two comparable groups of women were originally selected in the early 1960s, each consisting of about 31 000 subjects. One group was screened, using X-ray mammography and regular consultation with a doctor, whereas the other group was not screened (though no effort was made, of course, to prevent women in this group from seeking screening if they wanted it). Shapiro reports that there were fewer deaths from breast cancer in the years which followed among screened women who were over the age of 50 at the time the screening began (only women between the ages of 40 and 64 years were accepted into the study). The attractive conclusion is that screening not only detects breast cancer early, but that the death rates from this disease can thereby be reduced because treatment in an early stage is apparently more effective than treatment in a late stage in this age group.

Unfortunately, the benefits of breast cancer screening as reported in the American HIP study have not yet been confirmed by studies in other countries. In Britain the National Health Service is currently conducting a long-term study of screening for breast cancer in the hope that the advantages can be pin-pointed more accurately, and it does seem that although early detection and successful treatment of breast cancer could not remove the root cause of the disease in modern society, it might save some lives. But the exact number of lives is hotly debated.

Another problem with screening is a practical one. Most doctors agree that treatment for breast cancer helps the victim to live a better life, and in a minority of cases it is possible that it can actually cure the patient. But to screen all women over the age of 50 by X-ray examinations would require twice as many radiography centres and staff in a country like Britain as already exist. Even the most optimistic screening enthusiasts would not suggest that huge differences in the numbers of women dying from this disease could ever be produced by screening programmes and subsequent treatment. Although a range of different treatments are now being used for breast cancer, no approach has yet been shown to be markedly superior to another in terms of saving life (though it is more the question of preserving the quality of life which is often uppermost in the doctor's mind). It is not even clear whether some treatments actually cure the disease or just delay its development. If early detection does save lives, then there is something to be said for recommending women to examine their own breasts for lumps. Professor Michael Baum of London's King's College Hospital encourages this as he feels trials of all methods of combating breast cancer should continue to be practised, until it has been firmly proved that these are ineffective. Regular monthly self-examination costs nothing and does no physical harm, but women should beware of becoming obsessive about it. For the moment, breast cancer prevention, by minimising the risk factors I've already mentioned, seems undoubtedly better than cure.

Inherited risks

There is a slight tendency of breast cancer to run in families. What this probably means is that some women inherit from their parents a slightly higher than average susceptibility to the effects of a variety of things, such as diet and hormones, which are causes of breast cancer. So if the disease occurs in a particular family this by no means implies that the women in that family are all doomed to die from it. In fact it is the 'Western way of life' which seems to be a much bigger risk factor, and inherited susceptibility to the disease should not be regarded as a root cause.

But what are the facts? Since the 1940s it has been known that sisters and daughters of breast cancer patients have a between about two-fold and four-fold increased risk of getting breast cancer compared with similar women who do not have relatives so afflicted. This was established in studies by Dr O. Jacobsen in Britain in 1946 and several American studies, including that of Dr M. T. Macklin in 1959, where the number of breast cancer deaths among relatives of breast cancer victims was compared with the number expected on average in the population at large. More recently still, in *The Lancet* in 1983, Professor Malcolm Pike in Los Angeles and colleagues including Dr Ruth Ottman in New York confirmed this familial pattern of breast cancer. And Dr D. E. Anderson revealed in a series of scientific publications during the 1970s that the risk to relatives who have more than one affected relative is even greater: as much as eight times the average risk if, for example, a mother and a sister are both affected, with one of these having cancer in both breasts.

These facts are not very comforting to the female members of such families, but they do at least add statistical precision to their fears, and it is surely more helpful to be well informed about such matters than to be kept in ignorance. As well as this, the policy of screening is very much more acceptable in such high risk groups, and surgical treatment such as oophorectomy (removal of the ovaries) and even subcutaneous mastectomy (removal of the at-risk breast from beneath the skin) can be considered. Just as important, though, is the suggestion that families already affected by breast cancer should receive advice about the known facts concerning diet, hormones, pregnancy and other influences upon the risks of getting breast cancer. They should also be aware that the scientific evidence seems to suggest that influences very early in life generally and during adolescence in particular seem to be the most important. They could then take positive action to reduce their risks.

Some breast lumps lead to cancer – but most do not

It is also not very comforting to be told that certain types of benign (i.e. not cancerous) breast lumps also seem to be associated with an increased tendency to get breast cancer. One of the most recent studies of this relationship was reported in 1979 by Dr L. J. Coombes and Professor A. M. Lilienfield who followed the progress of more than 700 women found to have benign breast disease for up to 20 years. The risk of getting breast cancer was found to be three times greater in this group than among women without such breast disease. Again, not all breast disorders can be taken as a warning of possible cancer to follow in the future, and the great majority of women with benign breast disease do not get breast cancer. As with all of the other risk factors mentioned here, no absolute certainties are claimed. Any single risk factor should be taken as a warning only, and a combination of several risk factors in the same person as an even greater one.

Cancer of the ovary

Breast cancer is the commonest of the 'gynaecological cancers' in Western Europe and America, but cancer which begins in one or both ovaries strikes about one woman in 100 in these countries, often leading to death, and so is also alarming. There are two main types: that involving 'epithelial' cells, and the rarer form of the disease which involves the so-called 'germ cells'.

With germ-cell tumours, tissues within the ovary are affected which would normally be involved in forming eggs and taking part in the conception of a fetus. This form of the disease affects mainly young women and the causes are not at all clearly understood. But if this type could be diagnosed early enough and distinguished from the more common form of ovarian cancer (the epithelial tumour type which affects the surface layers of the ovary), it might easily be cured, according to experts such as Professor James S. Scott of the University of Leeds in England. The reason for this optimism is that another type of germ-cell tumour, testicular cancer, which often affects young men, reacts well to powerful anti-cancer drugs, and a drastic, but effective, cure can be achieved, so why not for female germ-cell tumours? One hope is that it may prove possible to spot germ-cell cancers of the ovary by using similar blood tests to the ones used in detecting testicular cancer.

As methods of preventing these tumours are so little understood, and as they seem to be (from the experience with testicular cancer) relatively curable, the recommendation at present is that medical research should be concentrated on better diagnosis and prompt treatment rather than prevention, an approach which has proved less rewarding for the more common forms of cancer affecting, in general, older people.

Some clues to the causes

Some clues do exist as to the causes of the more common type of varian cancer – the 'epithelial' form of the disease. In America, for example, it has been discovered that this is more common in white than in black women: so there may be an inborn susceptibility to the disease in white races. The disease is also much more common in old age and fairly rare in girls and young women. Also, this type of cancer seems to depend upon hormones in a way which is similar to the relationship between pregnancy, oestrogen and other hormones, and breast cancer. The key hormone as far as ovarian cancer is concerned seems to be the one called gonadotropin which is produced by the pituitary gland. High levels of gonadotropin seem to be related to high risks of epithelial cancer affecting the ovaries, but so far this theory has only been supported by experiments with mice; studies in humans have not been carried out. Pregnancy seems to protect against cancer of the ovaries, with one or more pregnancies cutting the risk in half compared with a woman who does not bear children. Since pregnancy causes a sharp fall in the levels of gonadotropin circulating in the blood stream, the connection between this hormone in humans and ovarian cancer seems to gain weight. In 1979, Valerie Beral and her colleagues at the London School of Hygiene and Tropical Medicine reported that trends in population records in England and Wales show that women giving birth to the greatest number of children had the lowest risks of developing ovarian cancer. This protection only applies to the more common epithelial type of ovarian cancer, however, and not to the rare germ-cell type affecting younger women.

There have been reports that taking the contraceptive pill can protect against ovarian cancer. Dr Muriel Newhouse and her colleagues in London, for example, report a near halving of the risk of this cancer among oral-contraceptive users. But in the *New England Journal of Medicine* in 1982 Daniel Cramer and his colleague in Boston, Massachusetts, reported their findings which showed that only women over the age of 40 experienced any reduction in the risk from ovarian cancer as a result of using the contraceptive pill. Among women under 40 there was no difference. Dr Cramer thinks it is therefore misleading to suggest a single overall risk benefit from using the pill and even feels that there is a chance that oral contraceptives might increase the risks of ovarian cancer because these tumours may start to grow in response to the oestrogen hormone in the pill. Nevertheless the many studies on pill effects conducted in America and Britain do collectively give evidence that the pill can have a substantial effect in protecting against ovarian cancer.

As with breast cancer, X-rays and other forms of atomic radiation increase a woman's risks of developing cancer of the ovary. Peter Smith and Sir Richard Doll reported in 1968 that radiation treatment (for another illness) in a group of women caused extra cases of cancer beginning in the ovaries, and other scientific studies, including following up the health of people exposed to radiation during the atomic bombing of Hiroshima, have confirmed their experience.

Womb cancer – caused by same factors?

Moving on to another women's cancer, the good news about cancer of the womb is that the form of the disease which is most commonly found (i.e. that affecting the endometrium, or lining of the womb) is usually cured by hysterectomy (removing the womb) when the disease is diagnosed early – as it normally is. The bad news is that it is common in the same high-risk groups of women who most often get breast cancer, being caused (as far as we know) by similar factors: a high-fat diet, being overweight, not having children and from using drugs containing oestrogen. For example, the use of hormone replacement therapy to remove symptoms of the 'change of life' and to combat the 'brittle bones' disease of osteoporosis discussed earlier has led to an epidemic of womb cancers in the United States, and doctors are now cutting right down on using oestrogen supplements for older women.

In Johannesburg, South Africa, Professor George Oettlé and Dr F. de Waard noted in 1965 that cancer of the womb was increasing among South African Blacks attending the Barawanath Hospital in Soweto, near Johannesburg. These racial groups had experienced almost no cases of womb cancer (as distinct from cervical cancer, where the cancer begins in the neck of the womb) at the time of a previous and thorough survey completed in 1960, and, after investigation, the scientists concluded that obesity was part of the reason for the increase. One explanation for this is that black women in South Africa now earn more money by working in cities such as Johannesburg and they develop Western diseases, such as cancer of the womb, as a result of a new, more affluent way of life.

Endometrial womb cancer is also commonly found among women who have high blood pressure, so it seems to be a typical 'Western disease' with causes ranging from overeating to delayed childbearing. The precise extent to which any of these projected causes contributes to a person's risks of getting endometrial cancer cannot be stated with any certainty, but it is reasonable to view with caution any aspects of our life-style which have been adopted relatively recently. Taking the contraceptive pill is an obvious example, although information on the risks of endometrial cancer following the use of the oral contraceptives have been reassuring so far. The American Cancer and Steroid Hormones (CASH) Study, still continuing, actually reports a protective effect, with women taking modern 'combined' pills (those containing both oestrogen- and progesterone-like drugs) being at only about half the risk of getting endometrial cancer compared with other women who use different methods of contraception.

A disease caused by doctors

The epidemic of endometrial cancer in the States which began in the mid-1960s and reached its highest point in 1975 (by which time the cause had been guessed) is a remarkable piece of medical history. It may go down as the most dramatic outbreak of an 'iatrogenic' cancer (i.e. caused by doctors) ever. A review of the epidemic was recently published by Dr Hershel Jick of the Boston Collaborative Drug Surveillance Program, who reports that 15 000 cases of endometrial cancer in America were caused by replacement oestrogen therapy between the years of 1971 and 1975 alone. Dr Jick admits that the medical world did not suspect that oestrogen therapy was the sole cause of this epidemic for some time because about one third of the women in the areas (such as the West Coast) where such therapy was most popular had hysterectomies after the menopause, thereby removing all possibility of cancer of the womb developing, and so the statistics were misleading. Also, it was the habit of physicians to prescribe oestrogens more intensively for women who had had hysterectomies than for women who hadn't. Consequently the effect of the largest doses in causing womb cancer were not measured. But now that the long-term results of such treatment on women who did not have hysterectomies have been analysed, it is clear that taking such therapy for over five years confers an extremely high risk of getting endometrial cancer.

Fortunately, the situation can be retrieved to some extent by performing hysterectomies on women who have taken, or who plan to take oestrogens for long periods of time, but it is nevertheless disturbing that a disease as serious as cancer could have been caused entirely by a new medical fashion. This is not to suggest that replacement therapy is without value; clearly it will remain an important option for treating certain female illnesses after the menopause. But in the light of the findings about this very specific cause of cancer, physicians everywhere are now a good deal more circumspect about making recommendations for its use in their patients.

Cancer of the cervix

In terms of trying to prevent cancer, breast and endometrial cancers share similar risk factors, and some of these also apply to ovarian cancer. The same is not true for cervical cancer which affects the neck of the womb, or cervix. About 4000 women contract this cancer in Britain each year and about half this number die. Yet it now looks as though *all* of these deaths could be prevented.

A cancer caused by infection

The success story of cervical cancer is one of the most satisfying in the whole field of cancer, both as far as understanding the causes is concerned and in terms of the improved success of treatment for cases which are detected early. It should be pointed out right from the start that the cervix is affected by a different type of cancer from the body of the womb. Unlike the other main types of gynaecological cancer it does not seem to be affected by hormones, and having a baby at an early age seems to give no protection. Most of the evidence about the sorts of women at risk suggests that cervical cancer is caused by a sexually transmitted infection, and although it is not altogether clear *which* microorganism is responsible for the disease, there are some likely candidates which I shall look at later.

It has been known for a long time that cervical cancer is very rare among nuns, and common in prostitutes. Also, women who have the disease are more likely to have married at an early age, more likely to have experienced sexual intercourse in adolescence, and to have had more than one sexual partner. As well as these clues which point towards the sex act as being involved in causing cervical cancer, it also seems that women who smoke are more likely to develop the disease. It is possible, of course, that it is just that women who smoke are also more likely to have intercourse at an earlier age than women who do not smoke, but it is also possible that the cancer-causing effect of tobacco smoke can affect the neck of the womb.

Changing sexual practices are thought to explain the changes in the incidence of cervical cancer over the years. For example, it has become less common in Europe and America since the earlier part of this century (though until 30 years ago cancers of the neck of the womb were not distinguished on death certificates from any other form of cancer affecting the womb, so the precise numbers of cases are not accurately known). This may be because prostitution is less common in these areas of the West now that sexual morals have been relaxed. The fact that prostitution is more common in South America where more strict sexual attitudes are still maintained suggests that infection from prostitutes may indeed be the cause. Similarly other differences in sexual practices could explain why it is quite common throughout most of Africa, and rare among Jewish people in Israel where prostitution is less common and monogamy the norm. It all points to the idea that prostitutes may harbour a pool of infection which is then spread by men to their wives or sexual partners.

Recently there has been a lot of interest in the importance of the 'male factor' in causing cancer of the cervix. Although the overall pattern of the illness suggests that it is a venereal disease, there are many patients who claim to have had only one sex partner. In view of this, a group led by Dr J. D. Buckley in Oxford, England, carried out a study of the husbands of women who were suffering from cervical cancer. It turned out that the husbands of the cancer patients studied had more often had sex partners other than their wives at some time during their lives than the husbands of other comparable women not suffering from cervical cancer (the comparison, or 'control', group). In *The Lancet* in 1981 the Oxford team therefore reported that their findings give support to the idea that cervical cancer is caused by an infection which in some cases is transmitted by husbands.

In 1982 Dr D. C. G. Skegg and colleagues in New Zealand, jointly with Professor Sir Richard Doll, put forward a fascinating hypothesis as to how the behaviour of men in different parts of the world and at different periods in history has affected the likelihood of women developing cancer of the cervix. In Latin America, the group suggested, cervical cancer is very common because men are expected to display 'machismo' and to be sexually experienced, whereas women are expected to remain virgins until married. It has been found that in certain South American countries where such values are held (rather as they were in Victorian Britain), men frequently use the services of prostitutes to obtain this experience. Because a large number of men have sexual relations with a relatively small number of prostitutes, the chances of the men becoming infected with the agent causing cervical cancer are quite high.

According to this hypothesis such societies are the most likely to suffer from high rates of cervical cancer, whereas the more 'permissive' societies, such as the United States, will suffer less since the men are likely to have sex with a much larger group of women in the community and the chances of their becoming infected are therefore smaller. On this hypothesis the safest communities as far as preventing this cancer is concerned would be religious sects and other groups where virginity in both sexes before marriage and sexual fidelity after marriage are practised. People who are completely celibate seem to be at no risk at all of getting the infection, whatever it is, which can cause cervical cancer in women.

Cancer of the penis linked to cervical cancer

Following a finding by Dr I. Martinez of Puerto Rico that penis and cervical cancers seem to be linked, an interesting study was carried out in New York State by Dr Saxon Graham and his colleagues at Buffalo, New York. They followed the health records of the wives of men suffering from cancer of the penis, which is quite rare in America and Europe. It was suspected that the cause of this cancer might also be an infection of some sort, and that the micro-organism causing it might also be involved in causing cancer of the cervix in women. Dr Graham and his colleagues found more cases of cervical cancer among the wives of these men than would be expected from the average national rate, which seems to support the idea that both cancers can be caused by the same infection.

In Britain, women born between 1911 and 1926 have for some time suffered from more cases of cervical cancer than average. It has been suggested that more of these women might have become infected with a sexually transmitted disease because their early adult life coincided with the Second World War when separation from husbands or sweethearts made it more likely that people would have more than one sexual relationship. Valerie Beral of the London School of Hygiene and Tropical Medicine reported a new study in 1974 confirming that the wives of men who travel a great deal in their work are more likely to contract cancer of the cervix than average, which underlines the importance of male sexual behaviour in causing this disease. This has been known since the 1930s and is also clear from American national records and statistics.

The pill implicated

A further risk factor connected with this form of cancer is, once again, the pill. In 1983 Professor Martin Vessey of Oxford discovered that cervical cancer is more common among women who take the contraceptive pill, and that this is apparently not because these women have more sex partners. This fact, and the association with smoking mentioned earlier, suggest that by no means everything is known about the causes of this disease. In his review of the subject, Daniel Cramer of the Harvard Medical School in the United States suggests that there are likely to be several different causes of cervical cancer, and that the full answer may not emerge clearly for some time.

Which infection is the culprit?

But what infective organism could it be that causes this disease? There has been a tremendous amount of interest in the possibility that a virus of the herpes family (similar to those which cause chicken pox, cold sores and shingles) is responsible. Herpes is certainly known to be capable of causing cancer in animals, but many cervical cancer patients have no obvious evidence of herpes infection, and most women with herpes do not get cervical cancer. There is also the possibility that herpes is only found among cancer patients because the virus tends to emerge from a dormant state in the body when something else affects the body's reactions. Just as cold sores appear on the lips when people get over-tired or when they suffer from a cold, so it is also possible that herpes is only found in the genital regions of the body because the cancer has stimulated it to come out of hiding, so to speak. In addition it may just be that herpes and cervical cancer are often found together in victims because both are connected with sexual promiscuity. It does not necessarily follow that the former causes the latter – the real culprit could be any one of a number of sexually transmitted diseases. The majority verdict at the moment is that herpes is probably not responsible.

Some new light was shed on the matter by Professor Harald zur Hausen of the Institute of Virology in Freiburg, Germany in the early 1980s. He and his colleagues have developed methods of looking for the molecular ingredients (the special DNA) of certain viruses in the cells of tissues taken from patients suffering from cervical cancer. As well as testing for the presence of the molecular parts of herpesvirus, the German team also looked for evidence of infection with genital wart virus (human papilloma-virus). Like herpes, wart virus infection is very common and has always been regarded as nothing more than a nuisance. But according to zur Hausen it may turn out to have a more sinister significance, in that it could be responsible, alone or in combination with another factor – perhaps an infection which has not yet been considered – for causing cervical cancer. His theory is that wart virus infection may continue the process of transforming cells from the cervix into cancerous ones after this process has been triggered by something else, such as another virus.

The advantage of tracking down the infectious cause or causes of this cancer is that it would then become possible to protect people from it by means of vaccination. The use of a vaccine may possibly embrace both protection against genital infections and against cervical (and perhaps penile) cancer. Unfortunately, it would take a long period of time to prove that any vaccine was effective in preventing cancer because of the lengthy period which seems to be necessary for most cancers to develop after the initial stimulus.

Early detection leads to cure

Because cancer is not one disease but many, it is not surprising that approaches to treatment and to prevention are quite diverse. Although doctors strive to cure all cancers, their attempts often fail with many of the common cancers as successful treatment is so difficult to achieve. Cancer of the cervix is not one of the commonest cancers in women, but neither is it the rarest. It is currently the seventh most common cancer among British women (if skin cancer is ignored), and about one woman in every hundred, on average, gets the disease. Encouragingly, of all forms of cancer it is one of the most susceptible to early detection and cure.

There seem to be several distinct phases in the development of cervical cancer. Firstly there is a period of abnormal cell growth, called dysplasia, which can be recognised by a skilled specialist as being different from normal cells. Dysplasia is not one universally recognised characteristic; there are discussions, and even disagreements, among medical people about what constitutes the condition. But there is a great deal of agreement about the fact that dysplasia can eventually (though by no means always) lead to cancer. If dysplasia is present it is detected in small quantities of tissue removed during the cervical smear test. If the affected tissue is then removed in a minor operation the women are cured and remain fertile.

The next stage in what is thought to be the growth cycle of cervical cancer is an abnormality called *carcinoma in situ*, which is a tumour that does not have the special 'invasive' quality of a cancer tumour. That is, it does not have a tendency to spread through the womb and into other organs. If this growth is removed, the chances of a cure are still 100%.

The third stage of the disease is called invasive cancer, and at this point the patient's life is threatened if the growth is not discovered and removed quickly. If the entire womb is removed (hysterectomy) at the early stages of invasive cancer, the patient's chances of a cure are still very good. So the medical opportunities for curing cervical cancer up to this stage are excellent.

The value of early detection and treatment was not accepted as definitely proven until recently. The problem was that once it was suspected, in the 1940s, that dysplasia and *carcinoma in situ* were likely to be followed by cervical cancer, it became impossible to put the theory to the test for obvious reasons. Any woman found to have these abnormalities would obviously want to receive medical attention to prevent the possible progression of the disease to actual cancer. Unfortunately this has made it especially difficult to prove conclusively that such treatment was a benefit since no 'control group' could be monitored, and until a year or so ago there were still dissenting voices who claimed that dysplasia and *carcinoma in situ* might not necessarily be forerunners of cancer, and might be quite harmless if left alone. The matter now seems to be proven, however, since the publication of work by statistician Dr Jack Cuzick of the Imperial Cancer Research Fund's Laboratories in London, who is among the scientists who have examined the death rates from cervical cancer in various countries. It is quite clear that in places such as Iceland

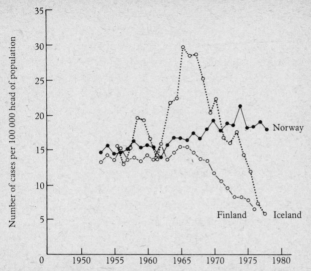

Fig 6 Annual incidence of cervical cancer in three Scandinavian countries from 1953–78. Large-scale screening programmes were instituted in Iceland and Finland in the 1960s and are continuing. In Norway no nationwide system for carrying out screening exists.

(Reproduced with permission of Hemisphere Publishing Corporation from 'Trends in the incidence of cervical cancer in Nordic countries' by M. Hakama in *Trends in Cancer Incidence: Causes and Practical Implications* (McGraw-Hill, 1982), edited by K. Magnus.)

and Finland where almost every woman receives a regular smear test, the death rate from this cancer has fallen dramatically. National screening programmes were instituted in these countries in the 1960s and by 1970 it is estimated nearly 90% of the female populations had been screened. Death rates from the disease in comparable countries such as Norway and Britain, where a very much smaller proportion of the female population receives a regular smear test to screen for cervical cancer, have fallen far less (*see Fig 6*). It is highly significant that in Iceland, where the age range screened is wider and the screenings more frequent, the cervical cancer rate has fallen the most.

The smear test

The smear test consists simply of removing a few cells from the neck of the womb so that they can be examined in a medical laboratory for evidence of dysplasia or *carcinoma in situ*. It is a quick procedure and quite cheap, so it could be carried out on all women quite easily. But it is not universally practised in, for example, Britain, where there is no national policy concerning such screening. As a result it is mainly the most well informed women who ask for regular smear tests and the most far-sighted doctors who suggest them. Less well educated women and those from poorer sections of the community are less likely to have this test – and they are the women most likely to be at risk of getting cervical cancer. This explains Britain's poor performance in cutting down the numbers of cervical cancer victims, as compared with Iceland and the United States. Obviously the question of choosing the best policy for detecting cervical cancer is a political one, but there is now little doubt among cancer scientists that deaths from cervical cancer could, in principle, become a thing of the past.

Under an ideal medical care system, every woman would be offered the smear test, or a comparable examination to discover the early stages of cervical cancer, at regular intervals – often enough to catch the disease before it has had time to progress. A test every three years for women over 30 is a basic rule often applied, but more frequent testing is recommended by some experts. Some guidelines were drawn up in Canada recently which suggest that women who are at the highest risk (such as those who have had many sex partners, smoke, who have had a sexually transmitted disease and who take oral contraceptives) should be tested every year. Women less likely to get the disease could be advised to opt for tests every two or every three years. But any woman who is worried about the possibility of getting cervical cancer should have the opportunity of being tested every year if she wishes. The more women know about this form of cancer and the certainty of cure if it is detected early, the more they will ask for such testing and the death rate from this truly curable cancer may one day disappear.

7 Infections that lead to cancer

In 1979 the world was taken by surprise with the outbreak of a form of cancer in America which until that time had been almost unknown in the West. In the medical journals of the 1980s there began a trickle, then a steady flow of reports about Kaposi's sarcoma, a cancer which is occasionally found in places such as Central Africa. The growing worry was that it was being diagnosed, for the first time, among young men in cities such as New York and San Francisco. It did not take long to discover that the victims of Kaposi's sarcoma, which is usually fatal, were mostly homosexuals, drug addicts, or haemophiliacs who have to receive many blood transfusions. What is more it soon became clear that this form of cancer was actually spreading from 'pockets of infection' in certain major cities in the United States and the nightmare of finding a form of cancer which can spread rapidly in the community and which particularly affects young people had begun.

Up until the 1980s infections did not seem to be the most worrying aspect of the detective story about the causes of cancer, but the epidemic of Kaposi's sarcoma has focused the attention of doctors all over the world on the fact that infections can suddenly become significant causes of this illness. Kaposi's sarcoma is one possible consequence of a new disease which has been named the Acquired Immune Deficiency Syndrome, or AIDS, to give it the usual abbreviation. This, briefly, is an illness where the body's natural defences against disease are greatly reduced. The result is that the victim falls ill with a variety of diseases, any one of which might have been the original infection which caused the syndrome. In 1984 Dr Robert Gallo of Bethesda, Maryland, announced that one virus in particular seems to be responsible for causing AIDS – a member of the group known as human T-cell leukaemia viruses. The discovery has given rise to the hope that this form of cancer may be eliminated if a vaccination against the virus which seem to cause it can be developed.

Cancers are not contagious

The emergence of AIDS has been just one dramatic illustration recently that cancer can be caused by infection. It should be said immediately that when people have contracted cancer itself they cannot infect another person with this illness. Cancer is not contagious. It should also be said that on present evidence only a very small proportion of cancers in the West are thought to be caused originally by infections. In the developing countries, however, the situation is more serious. A worrying fact about the evidence which now incriminates virus infections in causing certain cancers is that the particular types of virus which are principally suspected are very widespread, already infecting most people in the world. Viruses of the herpes family, which are already responsible for such common ailments as chicken pox, cold sores and shingles, are among the candidates. One herpes-type virus, the Epstein–Barr virus, causes infectious mononucleosis (popularly called glandular fever) in young adults, and usually infects children without causing any actual illness. So most people are infected with it at some time in their lives. Once infected with E–B virus, as with other herpesviruses, you are infected for life, mostly without it causing any illness. The worry is that under special circumstances these viruses may possibly help trigger cancer, for in the laboratory herpesviruses have proved capable of causing the disease in animals.

How virus infections can result in cancer is by no means well understood, but there is some evidence that it has to do with the natural 'machinery' within our genes. Research all over the world has shown that viruses are capable of inserting segments of new material into genes within living cells. Viruses of the herpes family, for example, may transfer some of their own 'gene material' into the genes of infected people and in this way could be part of the process leading to cancer.

Another way in which viral infections can cause cancer which is, in a sense, aided by man, is in transplant operations. Scientists such as Dr George Klein of the Karolinska Institute in Stockholm and, later, Dr Leo Kinlen and colleagues in Britain and Australia, have investigated the risk of contracting cancer among transplant patients. It has been found that there is a small increased risk of getting lymphoma in such cases. The reason for this is that transplant patients have to be treated with drugs to reduce their natural defences against foreign bodies, otherwise the donated organ might be rejected by the body's immune system. But this 'immune suppression' also reduces the body's defences against virus and other infections, and seems to increase the risk of certain rare cancers. The Epstein-Barr virus, which is present almost everywhere, may simply take this opportunity of multiplying in transplant patients and occasionally causing cancer. For this reason transplant teams in many centres, such as Mr Terence English's team at the Papworth Hospital near Cambridge, England, have adopted a policy of keeping the use of immunosuppressive drugs to a minimum and it is reassuring to note that among the heart-transplant recipients at Papworth Hospital there have been no cases of cancer. The need for watchfulness in this area, however, is immense.

Childhood cancer culprit identified

One interesting discovery of a form of cancer almost certainly caused by infection took place in Africa in the 1960s. Burkitt's lymphoma is a rare type of cancer which is almost exclusively found in Africa and a few other tropical regions. It was investigated by the Irish surgeon, Denis Burkitt (whose work on diet and cancer I described in Chapter 4), who worked for many years in Uganda. This cancer usually affects young children, often between the ages of five and eight, who come to the doctor with a growing lump or swelling in the jaws, or sometimes in the abdomen. It is the most rapidly growing form of cancer affecting humans, and can quite often be noticed to have enlarged within a single day. Without treatment the victims invariably die but it is encouraging that the disease responds very well to anti-cancer drugs. Denis Burkitt was fascinated by the pattern of distribution of this disease in Africa. It is limited to what is often called the 'lymphoma belt' which consists entirely of regions of high tropical rainfall and heavy infestation with malarial mosquitoes. As well as this, Burkitt discovered that even within this region there were areas where no cases were found. These were places which were more than 1500 metres above sea level. The evidence all pointed to the conclusion that this form of lymphoma must be related to rainfall, mosquitoes and the climatic effects of altitude – perhaps a result of an infection which can only be transmitted in the right conditions. Malarial infection was therefore thought to be involved, but mosquitoes cause malaria in many regions of the world, yet Burkitt's lymphoma occurs only in some of these regions. It was therefore thought that malaria could not be solely responsible. Eventually Burkitt's work centred around a search for a virus infection as the principal cause of this disease.

In 1964, Dr Anthony Epstein identified a virus from test-tube cultures of cells taken from Burkitt's lymphoma tumours. The virus was found to be a member of the herpes family, the one which is now called Epstein-Barr virus. The fact that this virus was then shown to be responsible for causing a very common illness in Western countries, namely 'glandular fever', justified the extreme scientific curiosity in a disease which until that point seemed to have no important significance in the West.

Malaria + Epstein–Barr virus = Burkitt's lymphoma?

All patients with Burkitt's lymphoma show signs of past or present infection with E–B virus, and the infection is usually more intense than in people who are infected but who don't contract the disease. It seems very likely that if this virus is responsible it can only cause Burkitt's lymphoma in the presence of a very heavy infestation of malarial parasites. This explains why high altitude protects certain communities even within the lymphoma belt, because in these areas populations of mosquitoes are greatly reduced.

It is still thought to be possible that the disease could occasionally be caused by other factors, as is typical of many cancers, but further research has continued to corroborate Burkitt's work. In 1978, for example, Dr Guy de Thé and his colleagues from the International Agency for Research on Cancer (based in Lyon,

France) published the results of a huge study in the West Nile district of Uganda. They collected blood samples from 42000 children up to the age of 8 and followed them up to see who developed Burkitt's lymphoma. They found that E–B virus infections precede Burkitt's lymphoma by several years.

In many ways the story of Burkitt's lymphoma is typical of the difficulties involved in making the definite link between infection and cancer. E–B virus is very common, so is malaria, and it still cannot be said with certainty that this combination of a virus and a parasite causes cancer. Many inhabitants (the majority in fact) of the lymphoma belt of Africa are infected by both these agents and do not get Burkitt's lymphoma which (like all childhood cancers) is very rare even in this region. But the thorough work of Burkitt, de Thé and the others has incriminated infection very strongly and more scientific work needs to be done in the laboratory or elsewhere to find out why most people so infected don't get cancer.

Liver cancer and infection

Liver cancer is one of the rarer cancers in Europe and North America although the secondary stages of many cancer growths do often spread to this organ. In South East Africa and part of West Africa, however, cancer of the liver is one of the commonest forms of the disease. (This is called 'primary' liver cancer to distinguish it from secondary growths in the liver from a cancer which has begun in another organ.) Earlier in the twentieth century, liver cancer was diagnosed more often in Britain than now, but this was probably because many cancers detected in the livers of patients were the secondary result of undiagnosed cancer tumours elsewhere in the body, so unfortunately we do not know the true incidence of primary liver cancer then. Today only one or two cancers out of every hundred in Western countries such as Britain and America are primary liver cancer, but there is a great deal of interest in this disease because it is thought to be caused chiefly by a virus infection. Promising vaccines are under development for the virus in question, namely the hepatitis B virus.

Again it has been international comparisons which have identified a virus as a possible cause of cancer. Scientists noted that the pattern of hepatitis infection throughout the world closely matched the pattern of primary liver cancer, although there are vastly greater numbers of people suffering the infection than the cancer. In Mozambique, for example, where liver cancer is the commonest type of cancer affecting young men, there is also a very great number of people infected with hepatitis – most of the population in fact. By contrast, in the United Kingdom, where liver cancer now seems to be very rare, only small percentages of the population are infected by this virus. There are about 200 million people world-wide who are chronically infected by hepatitis B, many of whom are not actually ill with the disease but harbour it in their bodies and pass it on, perhaps from mother to child.

The mere fact that hepatitis infection is commonest in places where primary liver cancer is also most common did not in itself prove that the virus causes liver cancer. In order to prove that the two are closely linked, scientists performed blood tests which can detect the presence of a 'label' on blood cells called the 'hepatitis B antigen'. This can indicate past or present infection with hepatitis B. As a result of this it is now known that liver cancer patients usually have strongly positive blood tests for hepatitis, but that these usually indicate a past infection, rather than hepatitis which is active and causing a viral infection at the same time as the cancer develops. In other words, it seems that after being infected with hepatitis, the virus can be harboured within the body for some time, probably for life. People so infected, but not showing any signs of illness from the virus, are called hepatitis carriers, and the virus can be passed from one person to another without any actual illness ever being obvious. But, although the infected people do not always develop the hepatitis disease, they may be liable to contract liver cancer as a result of the virus infection. A study in Taiwan carried out by Dr Palmer Beasley found that hepatitis B 'carriers' are 300 times more likely to get liver cancer than other people.

Other possible causes of liver cancer have also been put forward. For example, in tropical Africa, where liver cancer is common, the moist hot climate causes foods to become mouldy quite quickly. The *Aspergillus* mould on such food then produces the poison called aflatoxin which has been found to cause cancer in animal experiments (see Chapter 5). As a result it is strongly suspected as being another important cause of this disease. Drinking alcohol is another possible contributor to liver cancer and of these three candidate causes (hepatitis B virus, mould and alcohol) it is possible that more than one may need to be present in a person to produce the disease. Thus it is feasible that alcohol and hepatitis together form a 'carcinogenic' combination. Since Dr Beasley's work in Taiwan was reported in 1981, however, many people are now convinced that hepatitis B infection is the crucial factor and this has led to hopes of getting rid of both hepatitis and liver cancer altogether by eliminating the virus which causes them.

The promise of vaccines

At the London School of Hygiene and Tropical Medicine, Professor Arie Zuckerman is one of the principal subscribers to the idea that hepatitis is the main cause of liver cancer. He is chairing a World Health Organisation scientific group which has set itself the task of looking into the possibility of preventing liver cancer by vaccinating millions of people against hepatitis B infection in the high-risk areas. The WHO group members believe that four liver cancer cases out of every five are caused at least partly by hepatitis infection and that the priority is therefore to develop a vaccine against the virus which can be mass-produced cheaply. Vaccines have already been in existence since the 1980s but these are at present very costly to produce. Nevertheless they have shown that babies can be protected from the disease by vaccination shortly after birth and, if this technique were applied to all newborn infants in hepatitis areas, or to the infants of mothers identified (from blood tests) as carriers, then the chances are that liver cancer, currently one of the 10 commonest cancers in the world, could be sent along the road to extinction, along with diseases such as smallpox.

Professor Zuckerman and his colleagues in London are now working on a new, cheap 'second generation' vaccine, using only part of the hepatitis virus for injection to achieve immunity rather than having to take whole viruses, weaken them, and then inject them – a more complicated and expensive procedure. This means it may soon become economically attractive to mass-produce hepatitis vaccines since cost-saving could be achieved by growing the required viral ingredients inside bacteria which reproduce at a rapid rate, automatically manufacturing vaccine as they do so.

At the National Institute of Allergy and Nervous Disease in Bethesda, Maryland, Dr Geoffrey Smith and his colleagues have developed yet another method of mass-producing a hepatitis vaccine. This involves implanting proteins (units from which viruses are built) of hepatitis viruses into the cowpox (vaccinia) virus, normally used for vaccinating against smallpox. As methods of mass-producing cowpox virus are already in existence because of the need to protect people against the possibility of smallpox (even though the disease is now thought to be extinct), it may become possible to mass-produce the hybrid cowpox virus on which Dr Smith is working, thereby providing protection against both smallpox and hepatitis B simultaneously. Like Professor Zuckerman, Dr Smith is optimistic about the various possibilities for producing cheap vaccines to combat hepatitis in the future and this holds out a clear hope of significantly reducing the numbers of people who fall victim to liver cancer.

Nasopharyngeal cancer caused by virus

The exciting discovery of the Epstein–Barr virus, and the very strong evidence that it is one of the most important contributory causes of Burkitt's lymphoma, led to the idea (first investigated by Drs W. and G. Henle) that it might also be responsible for causing types of cancer other than this one. Patients with many other cancers are often found to be infected by more E–B viruses than average, although it has not been possible to distinguish whethe this is as a result of the cancer or whether the amount of virus present has played any role in forming the cancer or 'promoting' its growth in the first place. But a type of cancer has been identified affecting the upper airways and throat, called nasopharyngeal cancer, which does seem to be strongly related to the E–B virus. Every patient with nasopharyngeal cancer is found (by blood testing) to be infected with E–B virus and the intensity of the infection is related to the size of the tumour. As well as this the 'genetic material' (DNA) of the E–B virus has been found in cells from nasopharyngeal cancer tumours removed from patients suffering from the disease, which shows that genes from the virus have entered and become part of living cells which have turned into cancer cells.

Nasopharyngeal cancer is rare in most parts of the world but quite common in parts of China and South East Asia. It is also fairly common among Chinese *wherever they live*, so it seems this is one of the few cancers in which inherited susceptibility plays a big part. The tumour strikes mainly in adult life, whereas the infection with E–B virus almost certainly takes place long before. So it is a puzzle why the development of the cancer takes so long and why it happens in some people and not others. It has been discovered that nasopharyngeal cancer is more likely to develop among people who suffer from repeated attacks of illnesses of the upper airways, such as colds and 'flu. Such illnesses may be a con-sequence of infection with E–B virus as this can reduce the body's natural defences against a variety of illnesses (as it seems to do during an attack of 'glandular fever'). Dr Guy de Thé of the Inter-national Agency for Research on Cancer believes that there may be other contributing causes of this form of cancer but that the evidence incriminating E–B virus is nevertheless very strong.

Hodgkin's disease

A rare form of cancer affecting the lymphatic system, called Hodgkin's lymphoma, is yet another candidate cancer now being linked to E–B virus infection. It mainly affects young adults – often in their twenties – a few years after the age at which many people develop 'glandular fever', and it is more than twice as com-mon among people who have suffered from this disease than among people who never suffered any obvious illness as a result of the E–B virus. As with nasopharyngeal cancer, the intensity of past E–B infection, shown up by blood tests, is often higher among patients suffering from Hodgkin's disease. But not all patients with Hodgkin's disease appear to have had an E–B virus infection and the genetic material of this virus has never been found in tumour cells of Hodgkin's disease. It is therefore possible that both are there by coincidence, enjoying favourable circumstances. Fortunately, Hodgkin's disease can usually be cured by using powerful drugs capable of killing the cancer cells, so the outlook is by no means bleak.

Can leukaemia follow infection?

The causes of a range of cancers which affect the white cells of the blood, the leukaemias, are something of a mystery. It is definitely known that they can be caused by exposure to radiation but this probably explains only a small proportion of cases. Survivors of the atomic bombing of Hiroshima were found to be at a higher risk of developing leukaemia especially between five and 10 years after exposure to the radiation. Also, medical X-rays of unborn children and radiation treatment can cause this 'blood cancer' to develop. Yet most people suffering from the disease have not been exposed unduly to radiation and so many scientists have now come to believe that this family of diseases might also be caused by infections. In experiments it has been shown many times that animals, including mice, cats and monkeys, can develop leukaemia after being infected with a virus, but similar and presumably fairly conclusive experiments on human beings are obviously impossible.

First sign of human leukaemia/virus link

Although there is no proof yet that the commonest forms of leukaemia in man are caused by infection, a discovery was made in the early 1980s by Dr Robert Gallo and his colleagues in Bethesda, Maryland, of an infection closely linked to one very rare form of leukaemia known as adult T-cell leukaemia. Dr Gallo and his colleagues at the National Cancer Institute discovered a virus, now named human T-cell leukaemia virus, which seems to cause this special type of leukaemia found in certain parts of Japan and a few other places. He analysed the chemical structure of the DNA from the type of blood cells called T-cells (which give this type of leukaemia its name), and the striking discovery made was that in most cases the T-cell genes contained sections which are identical to sections of the genetic material of the newly discovered virus. It seems that the virus may be capable of entering these human blood cells and incorporating part of its genetic material into that of the human cell. This disturbance of the cell's normal genes (which under ordinary circumstances act like a 'master control centre', instructing the T-cell about what it should be doing and when it should reproduce itself) may be the trigger which causes the cells to become cancerous, reproducing themselves continually out of the body's control.

The practical value of Dr Gallo's work is that it should now be possible in theory to develop a vaccine to protect people against this type of cancer. It also proves for the first time that at least one type of human leukaemia can definitely be caused by a virus, and the special laboratory methods used to incriminate the virus are also being used widely among scientists to try to solve some of the basic problems about how all cancers begin at the level of an individual living cell. Although cancers caused by infections seem to be less common in Brtiain and the West than cancers due to other causes, there is a realistic, if distant, hope that such scientific work may one day yield some of the fundamental answers to the cancer problem. Dr Gallo's discovery in 1984 that a closely related T-cell virus is almost certainly responsible for causing AIDS and Kaposi's sarcoma is yet another important example of a particular virus emerging as a likely cause of a certain type of cancer.

The promise of all the scientific research on the infectious causes of cancer generally lies largely in the hope that vaccines will become available as soon as the particular viruses or other infectious agents causing particular cancers have been positively identified. This would make it possible to eliminate such cancers by mass vaccination programmes in the parts of the world affected. This hope is a long way off as yet, but the work on hepatitis is already very promising, and other possible infectious causes of cancer could well emerge in the near future.

8 Living with prudence

The human body is one of the world's most under-rated organisms. We have preconceived ideas about the capabilities of our minds and of our bodies, and for most people low expectations are a self-fulfilling prophecy. In one respect the human mind holds a great deal of power to prevent many diseases, including cancer: a power that lies in deliberately revising low expectations for health and deliberately choosing ways of fulfilling vastly higher expectations for enjoying all aspects of living – family life, work life, sex life, leisure life and everything else.

The approach to avoiding cancer should not be separated from the approach to avoiding other diseases or conditions which seem to be the bane of modern Western life: heart disease, stroke, bowel disorders, stomach ulcers, diabetes, piles, overweight, bronchitis, arthritis and so on. It seems not to be a co-incidence that 'prudent' measures aimed at lowering the risk of developing one of these 'Western diseases' also help to prevent most of the others. This is no more than some people would expect. Surgeon Captain T. L. Cleave, who in the 1940s and 50s pioneered many aspects of thinking about these so-called 'Western diseases' and how to prevent them, insisted that we do not fall ill because our bodies are weak, but because we misuse them. This, he thought, explained why many of 'our' diseases were almost totally absent from the developing countries, even among people who lived to the same age as in the West. Of course, such people suffer from other diseases, but in general these are related to social conditions, such as poor public hygiene which, it is hoped, will gradually be improved. A judicious 'return to nature', combined with the best of what modern hygiene and medical care have to offer, is now thought to be the way to add years, perhaps even decades, of healthy life to many Westerners.

The main hurdle to be overcome is the mental block we encounter when trying to persuade ourselves to look at life, death and disease in a different way. If everybody around us smokes like a chimney, drinks like a fish and eats like a horse and many of them live for three score years and ten, we tend to accept the 'status quo' rather than pushing for something better.

A 40 year-old lady, with a generous waistline, bopped energetically to an Elvis Presley single at a party I went to recently, and then sank herself, with evident relief, into a soft armchair nearby. Lighting a cigarette she remarked, while nodding towards an attractive 18-year-old girl, that when she was her daughter's age she used to dance all night and won several competitions for rock-and-roll dancing. 'But what can you expect at my age', she said. 'You have to slow down as you get older!'

It is difficult for most of us to realise just how wrong she was. Humans do not 'have' to slow down except in very old age; they should only be *forced* to do so by serious illness. One of Britain's leading marathon runners is a mother in her 40s. A recent Olympic double gold medallist in long-distance events is a man in his 40s. A 57-year-old friend of mine completed the famous 'Masters and Maidens' marathon in just over three hours – and there were older, faster runners ahead of him. The mistake most of us make is in assuming that such people are exceptional. There is no doubt that the ability to run marathons depends on physique and the efficiency with which the blood can absorb oxygen inhaled into the lungs. But fitness to dance, to make love, to drive all day without tiring, to eat and drink without feeling ill, and to enjoy (rather than endure) day-to-day activities is not limited to a small section of the community fortunate enough to have the right 'genes' which somehow give them a special ability to keep fit and alert. Most people could do a great deal more than they imagine, but are limited by habits so familiar they don't even realise they are dangerous and likely to lead to premature death.

The 'joy' of smoking

One obvious, and all too familiar habit is smoking – the single leading cause of cancer in Britain and many other countries, and principal ally of governments that don't like paying old-age pensions. There is no doubt that millions of people find smoking a great pleasure. And even if the pleasure itself is not obvious there is plenty of psychological pressure to attract them to the habit. Advertising, other smokers and even those who denounce smoking too vehemently as a dirty and even evil habit all help to convince the smoker that each cigarette yields a modicum of ecstasy, along with the milligrams of tar, carbon monoxide and nicotine. Fortunately millions of people enjoy the habit of inhaling ordinary air, free from tobacco smoke, and there are signs that the fashion of not smoking is already catching on – with the trend-setting higher social classes leading the way. A brilliant (but tobacco-addicted) cancer research scientist I talked to recently described how dramatically the fashion of not smoking has grown among some professional classes. At his research institution (in America) there are about 3000 scientists. When he first joined the establishment, at the beginning of the 1970s, about half of these were smokers. 'Today' he admits 'there are only three of us.'

In the 1940s smoking cigarettes was considered part of the transition from boyhood to manhood. It was as natural as breathing air. But fashions have changed. Among university teachers, doctors, scientists, lawyers and the leaders of business and industry, smokers are in a very noticeable minority. Smokers in such groups often decide to leave the packet behind when meeting with colleagues and re-stock their dwindling blood levels of nicotine on returning to the privacy of their own homes. To light a cigarette in company is becoming a deviant act. Smokers in offices are now frowned upon where in the past a smoke-laden atmosphere was simply regarded as normal.

There may, in the future, be legislation passed in many countries to limit tobacco smoking. Ten years ago this would have been almost impossible even to imagine. Today the non-smoking fashion is becoming so respectable that we can perhaps look forward to a time when 'No smoking' signs will be removed from public places, buses and railway carriages. Just as there is no longer any need for signs on buses asking passengers to refrain from spitting, so there will no longer be any need to announce that smoking is prohibited. It will become axiomatic even before laws are passed. One day it will seem astonishing to our grandchildren that non-smokers and smokers alike were forced during the middle years of this century to inhale other people's smoke in restaurants, cinemas, theatres, factories and offices – indoors almost everywhere. It will seem unpardonable that during the 1950s, '60s and '70s, no firm action was taken to cut the death-toll from lung cancer and heart disease caused by cigarettes, and that for many years non-smokers were ridiculed for objecting to tobacco smoke in the work-place or anywhere else.

One of the most striking differences will be the effect upon young people of the new attitude towards smoking. They already know that drugs such as cannabis may be dangerous because they have been banned by law, and even parents who still use such drugs themselves would not like their children to see them in the act. In the future tobacco use might generate a similar pattern of behaviour. Without being made completely illegal, cigarettes could gradually disappear from daily life. It would be quite clear to teenage children that only the 'dregs of society' allowed themselves to be seen smoking. Undoubtedly some children would nevertheless identify themselves with such an undesirable sector of the community, but most would prefer to imitate the vast majority of adults who would feel embarrassed to be seen smoking a cigarette. This trend is already beginning and is firmly established in some social groups, but it will need much more help from governments and the media before the 'non-smoking norm' is fully accepted by the masses.

What should smokers do?

Before that happy time is established, most of us have to put up with the fact that smoking is still common and is killing hundreds of thousands of us each year. Tobacco causes a third of all the deaths from all forms of cancer in America, more in Britain, and potentially as many as well over 40% of cancer deaths in both countries now that women have started smoking on a wide scale. So what hope is there for the smoker?

The principal hope is that he or she will quit. This brings a number of certainties. To begin with, smokers who have less than

Table V

Extra risk of various types of cancer incurred with obesity (calculated by Body Mass Index).

Type of cancer	Body mass index (weight in kilograms ÷ the square of height in metres)			
	25 (10–19% overweight)	27 (20–29% overweight)	29 (30–39% overweight)	31 (Over 40% overweight)
Endometrium (body of womb)	+ 36%	+ 85%	+ 130%	+ 442%
Cervix (neck of womb)	+ 24%	+ 51%	+ 42%	+ 139%
Gall bladder (in women)	+ 59%	+ 74%	+ 80%	+ 258%
Stomach (in both sexes)	+ 15%	+ 15%	+ 50%	+ 41%
Other cancers	Mostly a slight (up to 5%) increase of risk with obesity. Taken all together, cancers are 55% more common in obese women (i.e. BMI of more than 31) and 33% more common in obese men.			

(Data adapted from 'Variations in mortality by weight among 750,000 men and women.' by Lew and Garfinkel (1979), *Journal of Chronic Diseases* Vol. 32.)

about 10 years' moderate smoking on their record will almost certainly not get cancer as a result of cigarette smoking if they give it up for the rest of their lives. Most lung cancer victims are people who have smoked regularly for at least 20 years, so, allowing for the possibility that the cancer tumour may have been growing for 10 years before it was discovered (though this time estimate is a pure guess), it is reasonable to suggest that 10 years' smoking is unlikely to cause cancer. There are no guarantees on this point, however, so it is not recommended that anybody should embark upon the perilous project of becoming a smoker even if they then have the firm intention of quitting after 10 years.

Eat your greens!

There is evidence from Norway, Japan and the United States that even those who continue to smoke can reduce their likelihood of getting lung cancer by eating the sorts of food which contain the group of compounds, including carotene, referred to as vitamin A. The most important of such foods are green and yellow vegetables, including carrots, cabbage, broccoli, spinach, pumpkin and peppers. Liver, milk and 'multi-vitamin' pills also contain vitamin A and may help to reduce the risks of lung cancer, but as animal products contain fat, which is implicated in causing other cancers, on balance it is wiser to eat the vegetables. These should preferably be eaten every day, because any chemicals in them which might help prevent cancer from forming may not remain in the body for more than 24 hours.

Stay slim

All people, but especially smokers, should avoid becoming overweight since your cancer risks increase slightly when your bodyweight goes above average. The widely used formula for checking if your weight is ideal is to work out the body mass index, i.e. weight divided by the square of height. If you measure weight in kilograms and height in metres, this index should be in the range of 20 to 25 for men, and from 19 to 24 for women, according to most life insurance companies, and confirmed recently in the British Medical Journal by Dr John Garrow, an expert on the problems of overweight (*see Table V*).

Switch to low-tar brands

There is impressive evidence that switching to low-tar cigarettes reduces the risk of lung cancer, although there is absolutely no guarantee that it will reduce the risks of other smoking-linked diseases. On the evidence so far, low-tar cigarettes seem to be a little safer than medium- or high-tar brands, so any smoker who can enjoy low-tar brands should make the change.

Leave long butts

Leaving a long butt is almost certain to reduce cancer risks provided smokers do not compensate by smoking more cigarettes. The cancer-causing effects of smoking are dependent on dose, as well as the number of years you've been smoking. Cut down the number of cigarettes or the length of each cigarette smoked and you reduce the dose and cut your chances of getting cancer by the same amount. The most obvious piece of advice, therefore, is to cut down in any way possible (preferably to zero!).

How to cut down

Many smokers who are chemically addicted to nicotine cannot cut down easily. They automatically light another cigarette as soon as blood levels of nicotine and its related chemicals fall to a certain level because of a signal to the brain which operates in exactly the same way as our appetite for food. But some smokers are not addicted in this way – they smoke merely from habit in a variety of 'normal' situations. These people can cut down if they analyse the situations in which they are more likely to smoke and deliberately take action to avoid them.

One situation where most smokers tend to smoke more than at any other time is while drinking alcohol. 'A pint and a panatella' may sound an ideal combination if you are the manufacturer of either of these commodities, but if you want to avoid mouth, throat and gullet cancers you will treat this combination of smoking and drinking with a good deal of suspicion. With these three broad categories of cancer there is not much difference between cigarettes and other forms of tobacco smoking as far as triggering off cancer is concerned, and alcohol multiplies the effect. As well as this, the fact that people tend to smoke a great deal more during drinking sessions helps to keep the habit firmly rooted and makes lung cancer a much greater possibility. For these reasons smokers should try to avoid smoking while drinking. And by stopping drinking altogether they may find that the prospect of quitting smoking becomes a little easier to entertain.

Prepare for battle

Nobody should underestimate the difficulties of stopping smoking. Although there will always be a certain number of fortunate people who can give up easily, most smokers should be prepared for a battle. But the prizes are a much firmer prospect of living a longer, healthier life; feeling generally fitter; and having more money in your pocket! The benefits of quitting smoking are not confined to the young either, or those who have not smoked for very long. Older, long-term smokers are more likely to be on the verge of starting off a cancer in their lungs since (as I explained in Chapter 3) for this to happen it seems that a number of separate events need to occur over a period of time (rather like penalty points for driving offences building up to an automatic driving ban). By stopping smoking, even smokers of many years' standing could avoid receiving the final penalty point and so cut their risks of getting lung cancer.

Needless to say, efforts to give up smoking are made easier if encouragement can be given to the already growing fashion of not smoking in the community. Many smokers would welcome tougher legislation to restrict smoking because this would give them emotional support in their efforts to give up or cut down. A growing trend towards less smoking, coupled with new anti-smoking laws, would help many people to withstand 'peer-pressure' which has always made it more difficult for them to quit.

Eating with prudence

Apart from changing our smoking habits, the greatest untapped potential for avoiding cancer probably lies in changing our eating habits. In particular a move away from eating meat and other sources of fat which seem to be associated with some of the com-

monest 'Western' cancers is to be recommended. Fresh vegetables and fruits every day, and wholemeal bread and other 'high
fibre' foods also seem to be an important part of a 'prudent diet'
for avoiding cancer. What is more, most of the recommendations
for avoiding cancer by changing our diet are also likely to cut
down our risks of getting heart disease, strokes, and a good many
of the other familiar Western illnesses.

But eating patterns are often considered sacrosanct and any
suggestion of drastic change is regarded as being almost blasphe-
mous! This problem is compounded by a number of commercial
and political factors which make sure that the public eat what is
available rather than what would keep us free from cancer and
other diseases. It is ironical that the foods least likely to cause cancer and heart disease are intrinsically the cheapest to produce,
being largely of vegetable origin, whereas many of the suspected
cancer villains are the more expensive animal products. Unfortunately, however, one of the worst foods most incriminated by
'majority verdict' as a cause of both cancer and heart disease is
also very cheap because it is a by-product of the meat and dairy
industry. Fat added to a wide variety of popular modern foods is
generally devoured with gusto by an unsuspecting population in
sausages, pork pies, hamburgers, chips, ice cream, cakes and
countless other products.

Too many calories

Another risk factor is the amount of calories we consume. Sugar
and white flour in biscuits, sweets, cakes and white bread make it
possible for people to consume far more calories than are good for
them. Chocolate-coated glucose and sugar bars do not help people
work, rest and play any better than the same number of calories in
the form of fresh fruit or wholemeal bread. But they do make it
possible for them to consume easily far more calories than by eating the latter less refined, natural foods, and thus to run the risk of
'overconsumption', named by T. L. Cleave as the principal cause
of many Western diseases. In Chapter 4 I looked at the evidence
from insurance company statistics which show that overweight
people run a slightly higher risk of cancer than people of average
weight, and also at experiments with mice which have suggested

that too many calories might also have a dramatic effect in causing cancer in man. Such evidence clearly suggests that refined foods such as sugar and white flour should be avoided in favour of wholegrain foods and fruits which are lower in calories.

Freedom to exercise choice?

In general people are hardly aware that modern industry is forcing them to eat foods which are very different from the ones needed to avoid the Western diseases. White bread, processed foods, meat from 'fattened' cattle, fat-rich dairy produce, sausages and cooked meats containing added fat, these are all foods which serve the needs of efficiency and profit in the food production industry rather than being primarily designed for the very different requirements of preserving good health.

The food industry simply follows market forces and political pressures. So it is up to responsible people to make sure these forces begin to push in a more healthy direction. The question is: 'How long do we need to wait for indisputable proof about which foods cause disease before we can start taking such action?' At first sight the problem looks dauntingly complex. But when you begin to look at individual eating behaviour things become a great deal simpler.

Before going any further it should be made quite clear that the evidence about the formation of cancer in the body all points to the fact that only *long-term* hazards are likely to carry a significant risk of cancer. This is well worth knowing, because it means you can break all the 'rules' about prudent eating every now and again so long as you don't do so every day. A gluttonous binge on meats, sugar, cream and even strongly suspected carcinogens such as the Japanese favourite bracken fern, is hardly likely to pose a hazard if you restrict such behaviour to weekends or special occasions. But quite dramatic differences in cancer rates could be produced by relatively modest changes in eating behaviour over the long term, so from among the wide range of 'prudent' measures to be recommended, everybody can choose a combination which suits them individually. If you are addicted to full cream milk, for example, then don't worry: there are other foods you can forego in order to cut down on fats!

Start the day with prudence

Let's start with breakfast. In Britain and many other countries, an essential is the cup of tea or coffee. Through custom and habit many people add full cream milk. But those who take tea or coffee black not only taste the flavour of the drink more distinctly but also avoid the fat contained in the milk. An alternative strategy is to use skimmed milk. To cut down on potentially cancer-causing calories too, it goes without saying that sugar can also be dispensed with, again with a similar improvement in the flavour of your morning drink.

Cereal is highly recommended in a 'prudent' diet, but, again, the milk that often accompanies it isn't. The national campaign in Britain which encouraged people to 'drinka pinta milka day' is frowned upon by bodies such as the Coronary Prevention Group in London who believe that a pint of full cream British milk would contribute very significantly to heart disease unless most other sources of fat in the diet were eliminated. Apart from Dr Takeshi Hirayama's encouraging discovery that *in Japan* milk-drinking seems to help prevent stomach cancer, the bulk of the evidence suggests that we should drink less full cream milk to avoid cancers of the breast, bowel, womb and various other parts of the body. The answer? Substitute skimmed milk on your cereal, or dilute the milk with water.

The choice of breakfast cereal is also important. The ones which are clearly labelled as consisting of 100% wholegrain will provide more 'dietary fibre' than other cereals, and this could help reduce a whole range of disorders relating to the bowel, including bowel cancer in the long term, and constipation and piles in the short term.

To get over the problem of satisfying a 'sweet tooth' without vastly increasing your calorie intake by adding sugar to your breakfast cereal, try dried fruits such as currants, raisins, and dried apricots, bananas and prunes. T. L. Cleave suggested this to me since he acknowledges that nature has given many of us a liking for sweet things, which before the industrial age was satisfied by eating fruits and berries. To derive sweetness from these foods we have to eat a large amount of the fibre they contain too, which automatically protects us from overdoing the calories since there simply isn't enough room in our stomachs to overconsume. It is also comforting to know that by eating natural fruits we can allow our gluttonous natures free reign – no medical problems of any magnitude have yet been reliably blamed upon excessive fruit-eating!

So, now that you've taken a cup of tea (preferably without milk), eaten a dish of wholegrain breakfast cereal with skimmed milk and dried raisins, the next course needs careful consideration. The traditional British dish of eggs (note the plural) and bacon, served with sausages (also plural) and fried tomatoes is a bit risky if eaten daily unless you are also careful to eat little in the way of meats and fat during the rest of the day. As with all matters relating to the 'prudent diet', no foods should be forbidden, but there is a great deal to be said for eating such traditional British fare on Sundays only. The problem, of course, is the fat content of such a dish. To make matters worse still, some establishments (particularly transport cafés) serve this dish together with white bread and butter – adding to the calories *and* to the fat. You may even get *fried* bread! To dissuade you from scoffing such fare on a daily basis then, here come the facts and figures.

To prevent heart disease (the biggest killer of all Western diseases) the Coronary Prevention Group recommends that no more than one egg a day should be eaten. Two eggs daily, plus bacon, sausages (which usually contain a huge amount of fat) and fried bread is probably a recipe for early heart disease. According to the US National Research Council's recommendations, published in its report on *Diet, Nutrition and Cancer*, the average level of 40% of calories in a typical meal being in the form of fat is far too high. The traditional British breakfast plate usually has far more than 40% of its calories in the form of fat and so should be considered extremely hazardous by those wishing to follow a prudent diet.

The hazard would only have a chance of causing cancer, however, if this level of fat intake were maintained every day for many years. And extra fat at breakfast could be balanced by low-fat meals during the rest of the day. So those of us who adore bacon and eggs can eat them from time to time without anxiety, particularly if the eggs are poached and the bacon grilled. But there's still a lot to be said for doing without the sausages!

The prudent eater would have wholemeal toast to conclude the British breakfast and spread it only thinly with butter or margarine. He or she would choose a jam made without added sugar, which had been sweetened entirely from the sugars contained in the fruit and set with natural pectin, instead of the ordinary marmalade or jam available in shops which often contains an extremely high percentage of sugar.

Continue as you've started

When it comes to eating the main meal of the day, one of the first things to say is that if you have eaten a full traditional British breakfast, then that *was* your main meal! Lunch and dinner should be frugal affairs after such a start to the day. The fact that it is considered normal to eat a two-course lunch and perhaps a three-course dinner as well may help to explain the incidence of many Western diseases and give some clues as to the reasons behind Britain's high rates of bowel and breast cancer.

However, the quantity of food you eat is one potential hazard which becomes less dangerous if the foods eaten are rich in fibre. This does not only mean wholemeal bread, high-fibre breakfast cereals, or bran. There are many different high-fibre foods, and among the most under-rated are the legumes. Beans, peas and lentils were formerly very popular in many Western countries, but with the increase in affluence they have been replaced by meat. Legumes are very low in fat, provide adequate protein and have a very helpful effect on bowel action.

A prudent eater would therefore take meat no more than once a day, and even then in small quantities: a few ounces of steak – not the 8- or 12-ounce slabs served in popular steakhouses. Large steaks may be appropriate to restaurants where most people will eat occasionally rather than on a daily basis. But such helpings of meat are anything but appropriate at home, in the works canteen, or in the staff restaurant. Meat itself has been related to an increased risk of some types of cancer and is also, of course, a source of fat. So on both of these counts meat should be restricted. To fill the gap, the legumes offer many delightful alternatives.

Most people think of beans and lentils as plain foods, but this is mostly because they are traditionally served (in the West at any rate) as an adjunct to the meat dish, and all the chef's culinary skills are devoted to the latter. But there is no reason why these same skills should not be used on the humble bean. When legumes are prepared with red wine, garlic, herbs and exotic vegetables, they taste every bit as delicious as meat prepared in the same way. By focusing attention on the legumes, and excluding meat from the meal, gastronomic enjoyment can be achieved at the same time as great reduction in fat intake. (Even lean meat, incidentally, contains a substantial amount of fat.)

The task of producing low-fat recipes which are also attractive to the average Westerner has occupied the minds and taxed the ingenuity of nutritionists for several years now – ever since it became clear that less fat in the diet would mean less heart disease in the community. Now that the American report *Diet, Nutrition and Cancer* has also recommended low-fat diets as possibly the most important nutritional step to take for preventing cancer, there is even more reason to seek acceptable meals which contain little fat. Substituting legumes for meat is a very sound way of achieving this, and you can make the substitution without the meat being missed. In fact, the main reason we eat meat currently is to keep livestock producers in business. Today there is no nutritional argument left to defend the huge quantities of meat and fats in the typical Western diet.

While on the subject of eating peas, beans, lentils and other legumes in generous quantities, one demon should be laid to rest. Many people worry that eating beans leads to socially unacceptable quantities of 'wind' in the bowels. This is a point upon which some reassurance can be given. To begin with it is quite true that when a person who normally eats food containing very little fibre (such as cheese and white bread, cakes, milk, meat) subsequently eats beans, the result is the production of flatus. But if fibre-rich foods (including wholemeal bread and cereals, fresh fruits and vegetables) are eaten daily as well as legumes, there is less 'wind' and, perhaps more importantly, no unpleasant odours because certain bacteria associated with the modern refined diet are present in the bowel in much smaller quantities.

Another reason for considering legumes as a good food to substitute for meat stems from a body of work carried out first of all in London and Oxford in England, and now principally at the University of Toronto under Dr David Jenkins. This has shown that a diet which is rich in legumes has many advantages for diabetics, since it slows down the rate at which blood glucose levels rise after a meal. It also reduces the concentrations of certain types of cholesterol fats (lipids) in the blood. On the principle expounded by Cleave and Burkitt (discussed in Chapter 4) it is reasonable to suggest that a diet which is beneficial for one Western disease (namely diabetes) is likely to be appropriate for people at risk from other Western diseases too. No absolute guarantees can be given, but the evidence all points to the advantages of including more legumes in your diet which surely outweigh any minor disadvantages. It is simply up to you to make the choice.

The recommendation mentioned earlier in this chapter to smokers to eat more fresh vegetables for their protective effect also applies to non-smokers, of course. Just about everything commonly available in this modern world of refrigerated transport which now gives most people in industrial countries a superb choice of freshly grown crops is to be recommended. Cabbage, pumpkin, spinach (fresh – not canned, despite what 'Popeye, the Sailor Man' would recommend), Brussels sprouts, courgettes, broccoli, cauliflower, carrots, red and green peppers are all ideal for daily prudent eating. All of the root vegetables, including potatoes, parsnips, swedes, turnips and more exotic ones such as yams and sweet potato are also highly recommended because (among other things) they help you to cut down the proportion of fat in your meals. During the 1950s such vegetables were held in low esteem by slimmers because the nutritional text-books classed them as carbohydrates no different from sugar and white flour, and therefore another source of calories. But there is a big difference between carbohydrate in the form of sugar or white bread, and carbohydrate in the form of root vegetables. Fresh root vegetables are absorbed more slowly in the gut and, because of their high fibre content, help to fill the stomach and so prevent us from over-eating. A generous helping of plain boiled potatoes is very good for slimming because it helps you to eat less fat which is mainly contained in the meat and gravy of the typical Western meal. So root vegetables help make it possible for people to keep the fat content of an average meal well below the 40% level which the American report on diet and cancer considered to be dangerous.

In short, if you include a variety of fresh vegetables in all your main meals, you will be reducing your risks of developing cancer in three ways. You will be consuming a small extra amount of dietary fibre (which, perhaps importantly, is different from the type of fibre in your breakfast cereal and wholemeal toast) and this will help any potentially cancer-causing substance in the food to pass through the gut quickly. You will benefit from any preventative effect the vegetables have, whether this be the result of the vitamin A in them or something else. And, finally, you will be satisfying your appetite with foods that we are fairly sure are harmless and so will eat less of those which we are fairly certain are harmful, such as fat.

The ideal main meal

To summarise: your main meal of the day should have at most a *small* portion of meat (a few ounces only), or in place of the meat a legume-based dish, with plenty of root vegetables to provide calories in the form of slowly absorbed, *complex* carbohydrate (not simple, quickly absorbed carbohydrate like sugar), together with several other different vegetables. A ratatouille-type mixture, for example, of chopped courgettes, leeks, tomatoes, red and green peppers, aubergines, celery, onions and garlic, cooked with a tablespoonful or so of olive oil and half a glass of white wine (this quantity of fat and alcohol on its own does not constitute a cancer hazard) makes a delicious and yet very prudent accompaniment. Commercially manufactured sauces and relishes are *not* a recommended addition to such a meal, since most are made with a great deal of sugar.

Salads, of course, are highly recommended, especially when not drowned in high-fat mayonnaise or blue-cheese dressing. There is a suspicion that the present day reduction in the incidence of stomach cancer in the USA has been brought about in part by the American predilection for side salads with every meal (coupled also with the magnificent availability of fresh fruit in the United States). The many different varieties of lettuce contain indoles, which are thought to inhibit the formation and growth of cancer tumours, and most fresh salad vegetables contain substances such as vitamin C which are thought to help prevent stomach cancer, possibly by stopping the formation of carcinogens such as nitrosamine in the stomach. There appears to be no known danger in eating salad with every main meal! On the contrary, there is every indication it will do you good.

A final word on the subject of vegetables – the anti-cancer properties which they are thought to possess are probably due to the presence of chemicals such as vitamins in these foods. Such chemicals are delicate formations of atoms and may easily be destroyed by cooking. In view of this there is a lot to be said for taking every opportunity of eating raw vegetables. Many children are delighted to be given a fresh young raw carrot to chew, and if they get into the habit of taking snacks in this way, rather than by eating sweets or chocolates, they are more likely to avoid illnesses in the future. By the same token, when you do cook vegetables they should be cooked as little as possible. They should still be crisp and crunchy when they reach your plate, not limp and soggy with all the 'goodness' having been poured down the sink along with the water they were boiled in.

Moving on to dessert, one of the best (and most convenient) approaches is to provide unlimited fresh fruit to finish the meal. In this way sweetness is available in a form of food which contains dietary fibre and which also contains the recommended vitamin C in its natural form. Probably the very worst type of dessert is a creamy, sweet cake such as Black Forest gateau. This represents the epitome of what not to eat after a rich main course. But there is at least some salvation for those who are addicted to such excesses: if you can only persuade your appetite to refrain from eating such high-fat dishes *every* day, you can quite literally have your cake and eat it. Anybody who eats a fat-laden meal once a week, but eats prudent low-fat dishes the rest of the time is probably most unlikely to suffer the feared consequences of the typical Western diet.

Chips with everything

The huge growth of 'fast food' chains throughout the Western world poses another problem to the prudent eater. Hamburger and chips, fish and chips, deep-fried chicken and chips, washed down with enormous milk shakes made from full cream milk and plenty of sugar, are probably quite harmless when eaten *occasionally*. But there are huge commercial pressures, particularly from television advertising aimed at the young, which are persuading more and more people to eat these foods *every day*. It is creditable that many of the fast food chains have pioneered computerised efficiency, cleanliness and excellent staff relations which have made their products cheap and fun to eat. But this very efficiency has made competition from other types of restaurants difficult and the 'image' promotion has been so successful that many children now will not willingly eat anything else.

This is particularly worrying since most of the dietary influences on cancer (and probably on the other 'Western diseases') seem to exert an effect early in life, so it is important to establish prudent eating habits among children, which they will hopefully continue for the rest of their lives. Even if they change these habits after leaving home, there is still a good chance that any potentially disease-causing eating patterns they adopt in adulthood will cause less harm then. A great deal of evidence suggests that factors which cause two of the commonest cancers in Britain – stomach cancer and breast cancer – operate mostly at a very early age, so prudent eating in childhood could make a great difference to our cancer risks.

Because most 'fast foods' include plenty of fat and low-fibre, easily absorbed carbohydrates like sugar and white flour, they are quite the opposite of what the Royal College of Physicians and the Coronary Prevention Group in Britain would recommend for avoiding heart disease, and equally inadvisable, according to the American National Research Council's report, for avoiding cancer. The art of eating prudently depends on regularly including fibre-rich low-fat wholefoods and fresh vegetables and fruits in your meals, but allows an occasional indulgence in almost any other dish. But to make a habit of eating junk foods every day is almost certainly asking for trouble. Certain groups of people, such as athletes, dancers, professional football players and others indulging regularly in very vigorous exercise, may be able to take more liberties than the rest of us (although this is not proven). But even very active people would be well advised to follow prudent eating patterns if they want to lead a long and healthy life.

Exercise and cancer

The whole question of exercise and its role in preventing a range of different illnesses is a controversial one. Most doctors will advise their patients to take exercise, but they mostly admit that there is not much scientific documentation about the health benefits this produces. As far as heart disease is concerned, Professor Jeremy Morris of the London School of Hygiene and Tropical Medicine is one of the few scientists who have investigated the effects of vigorous activity, such as swimming or jogging, on our chances of dying from a heart attack. He is convinced that exercise protects. Other scientists have found that exercise alters the amounts of certain cholesterol-type fats in the blood in a way which is likely to reduce the risks of heart disease, and a large number of investigations have shown that exercise improves the circulation of blood. As far as cancer is concerned no similar studies have been carried out, but there are reasons for believing that exercise may help prevent some forms of this disease.

Fitness fights fatness

For one thing, it is very difficult to take vigorous exercise such as marathon-running and be overweight. Information from life insurance companies, recently reviewed by Dr John Garrow of the Northwick Park Hospital in London, suggests that deliberately losing weight can reduce the risks of a variety of diseases, including cancer. The usual approach to losing weight is to suggest dieting. But this may not have any effect on a person's metabolic rate which, if it is lower than average can be the root cause of their being overweight. Prudently increasing exercise (by beginning with a little, and gradually – over weeks and months – building up to more vigorous exercise) can at least help the body to burn off excess calories. If the slimmer feels even more hungry as a result, then eating a whole range of prudent foods (low in fat and sugar) will probably not add extra bodyweight. Even if an active person does not actually lose weight, he or she is more likely to have bulky muscles than bulky fat tissues in his or her body, and, according to the theories of Dr de Waard in Holland, the replacement of fat by muscle is almost certainly a good thing for reducing the risks of breast cancer and other types of cancer strongly linked to fat in the body as well as fat in the diet.

A comforting message for people who find it impossible to lose weight is that people who are 'genetically fat' may not be so much at risk from cancer and heart disease as people who are fat because of overeating. If a naturally plump person takes regular and quite vigorous exercise and keeps to a prudent diet, there are reasonable grounds for expecting that this pattern of behaviour will protect against the Western diseases, including cancer, irrespective of whether he or she loses any weight. Fitness and wise eating are probably far more significant in avoiding illness than any absolute measure of fatness.

Alcohol causes cancer

The 1981 report by Doll and Peto to the American Office of Technology Assessment attributed 3% of all human cancer deaths to the drinking of alcohol in all its various forms. A large proportion of this figure seems to be caused by alcohol in combination with other cancer risk factors, such as smoking or hepatitis B infection, but in addition to the obvious risks which stem from regular alcohol drinking, it is also clear that alcohol is a source of calories lacking in dietary fibre. Such a readily absorbable form of 'food' can obviously contribute to 'overconsumption' and obesity. Regular drinking also makes it more difficult to take other prudent measures, such as giving up smoking and taking more exercise, so there are plenty of reasons for being careful about drinking. Modest weekend drinking is preferable to daily drinking, even in small amounts, despite some evidence that regular small amounts of alcohol may help prevent heart disease and gallstones by reducing certain 'cholesterol' concentrations in the bile and blood. Dr Kenneth Heaton of Bristol, England, recently found that half a bottle of wine a day brings this benefit, though he does not suggest that people begin drinking this amount of alcohol. He believes that a smaller amount may produce the same benefits to the blood and biliary fat (or 'lipid') levels, and that rather than advising people to drink, the message should be to reassure those who already drink that small quantities of alcohol may do some good as far as certain illnesses are concerned. But most of the evidence suggests that it gives no protection against cancer.

Sex and the prudent life-style

Because cervical and penile cancers are now thought to be caused by sexual contact, it is obviously even more advisable than ever to take steps to stop the spread of sexually transmitted infections in the community. Although monogamy would be the ideal type of sexual relationship from this point of view, there is the risk that societies promulgating such norms would evolve 'double standards'. As happens in many Latin American countries now, men would seek prostitutes before marriage to learn about sex and then marry virgins. This might create an intense 'pool of infection' among the prostitutes which, if uncontrolled, would spread widely among the men in the community who would then infect their wives after marriage.

For the present, the existence (in more favoured regions, at least) of good health care and increasing recommendations to women at highest risk to have smear tests for the early detection of cervical cancer give some safeguards. In addition, the use of barrier contraception, rather than the pill or coil, can give individuals more protection against infection and therefore possibly cancer, and ultimately it is hoped that vaccines will be developed to give people immunity from the infections suspected of causing the disease. Cervical and penile cancers are generally more common among communities where hygiene is poor, so it is possible that washing the genital areas gives some protection against transferring infection. However, the suggestion that circumcision helps prevent cervical cancer has been refuted. There seem to be other factors at work in communities practising circumcision which explain the lower rates of these cancers noted among them.

Manipulating pregnancy and hormones

The incidence of the so-called 'gynaecological' cancers (i.e. of the breast, womb and ovaries) seems to vary a great deal according to life-style. But the risk factors which can most easily be changed are already known to doctors and women alike. Hormone replacement therapy to help cope with the effects of the 'change of life' or to halt the bone-loss disease, osteoporosis, is now limited to those women whose need for treatment justifies the additional risk of womb cancer which it carries.

The contraceptive pill is also under scrutiny as a possible cause and, even though it may in the end turn out to be harmless, women under the age of 25 should still think twice before taking it for long periods of time. It may increasingly come to be regarded as a 'stop-gap' form of contraception because of the possible cancer hazard involved in its long-term use, and be prescribed only until other forms of contraception can be arranged. Women over the age of 35 who smoke are already discouraged from taking the pill because of the effect it has in helping to cause heart disease, so there seems to be a decreasing age range of women for whom this convenient form of contraception is acceptable on medical grounds. It may turn out that some formulations of the pill will affect cancer rates, and others not. The field of understanding of the cancer risks of the pill is wide open at the moment, so the prudent approach would be to seek other forms of contraception, such as barrier methods, until the questions have been resolved.

One of the biggest influences on breast cancer risks and also upon the likelihood of developing ovarian or womb cancers is the condition of pregnancy. An early first pregnancy seems to protect against these diseases and this probably goes some way towards explaining the low breast cancer risks which exist in developing countries. In the West it is widely held to be impractical to advise women to have a baby just in order to cut their chances of getting breast cancer, but a positive step which *could* be taken would be to reduce the extreme difficulties connected with the work place which deter women from starting a family early even if they wish to do so. One of the reasons for rising breast cancer rates in the West is that women are forced to delay pregnancy, whether they want to or not, in order to be able to pursue a career. Those who interrupt their working life to have babies or, more significantly still, their student days, risk losing opportunities in the job market-place which under today's systems in many countries will not arise again. This is quite unfair on grounds of equality of the sexes, quite apart from the effect it has in increasing breast cancer risks. Many women might, of course, want to delay pregnancy for other reasons too, but it is wrong that they should be forced to do so by social circumstances. Clearly it is not only job opportunities, but also the growth of the so-called 'consumer society', which has influenced decisions about the timing of pregnancies. There is a firm belief among young couples nowadays that material goods are essential to a happy life and earning money to pay for these therefore often takes precedence over starting a family. What is needed is more *real* choice for women as to when to bear children. Some would certainly decide to have babies earlier if the circumstances were more convenient, and this would reduce (to some extent, depending on the numbers of such women) the rates of breast cancer.

Shun the sun

Exposure to sunlight is one of the commonest causes of cancer, but as this usually only leads to common skin cancer, which is almost always curable, there is no need to fear the sun's rays on that account. A more sinister possibility is that sunbathing may cause the rarer, fatal form of skin cancer known as melanoma. For this reason sunbathers should moderate their exposure.

Cut down on X-rays

Another step you can take to avoid cancer is to avoid *unnecessary* X-ray examinations. The work of Peter Smith of the London School of Hygiene and Tropical Medicine and Sir Richard Doll of

Oxford University has shown that humans can receive quite large doses of radiation and not get cancer. But they also found that the enthusiasm for using X-ray therapy earlier this century for certain diseases (the back condition called ankylosing spondilitis was one, in particular) caused a small number of cancers among the many people who received such treatment. Because present day X-ray examinations (rather than treatment) use *much* smaller doses of radiation, it is unlikely that these would cause cancer. But a whole series of X-ray examinations would pose a proportionately greater risk. Pregnant women should certainly never be X-rayed unless there is a very important reason, because a fetus seems to be very much more susceptible to the cancer-causing effects of radiation.

Similarly, airline passengers take a small risk when they take a jet flight above most of the earth's atmosphere where cosmic rays are more intense and therefore more likely to cause cancer. This is one of the reasons why pregnant women are sometimes advised not to fly. But to get worried about a dental X-ray, for example, whilst at the same time continuing to smoke cigarettes would be quite ridiculous. Medical and dental X-rays are known to pose very little cancer risk (as long as the right precautions are always taken). Smoking, on the other hand, is the known cause of many millions of cancer deaths all over the world.

What should you do first?

It is very important to get our priorities right. Smoking is the biggest cause of cancer in the Western world, and the incidence of lung cancer is also now rising in countries in the Third World where the habit is becoming popular. Food may play a very big role in causing Western cancers too, with alcohol having a small but significant bit part in the play. Not having a baby at a young age helps cause many (perhaps the majority) of 'female cancers', except for cervical cancer, which seems to be caused entirely by infection through sexual contact. But after these major causes, the remaining hazards, including certain occupations and forms of medical treatment, excessive X-rays, exposure to certain industrial products and agricultural chemicals, and perhaps some

Table VI Breakdown of percentage of cancer deaths attributed to different causes.

Cause	Estimated percentage of all cancer deaths	Range of acceptable estimates
	%	%
Tobacco	30	25–40
Alcohol	3	2–4
Diet	35	10–70
Food additives	less than 1	−5*–2
Reproductive and sexual behaviour	7	1–13
Occupation	4	2–8
Pollution	2	less than 1–5
Industrial products	less than 1	less than 1–2
Medicines and medical procedures	1	0.5–3
Geophysical factors (eg sunlight)	3	2–4
Infection	10	1–?
Unknown	?	?

* Allowing for a possibly protective effect of antioxidants and other preservatives.
Data from *The Causes of Cancer* (OUP, 1981) by Doll and Peto.

food additives and forms of pollution, are probably far less important (*see Table VI*). Cancer scientists Peto and Doll believe that in America (the country for which their precise calculations were done) about two thirds of all cancer deaths are caused by tobacco and diet, so the other cancer hazards individually make a much smaller contribution to our risks and therefore offer less scope for preventing cancer among large numbers of people.

However, for individual people in particular situations, minority causes of cancer can obviously be very important. For example, although great improvements have been made in the working conditions for most employees in modern industries, it is as well to be aware that long-term exposure to *any* industrial product which has not already been exonerated as a cause of cancer should at least be regarded with suspicion. The known facts about asbestos and the entire range of proven industrial carcinogens should serve as a warning to those who handle such products –

health regulations should be observed and improved upon if there is any cause for concern.

Although the consensus is that most human cancers are potentially preventable, it is important to realise that no absolute guarantees can be given. Every circumstance which seems to produce cancer gives only a *risk* of cancer to individual people, no certainty. Each risk you take is like playing Russian Roulette, but with hundreds of empty barrels in the revolver. You may get away with taking a good many cancer risks and never get cancer. On the other hand a few unfortunate individuals may get cancer as the result of being exposed to a very small extra risk. What is clear, however, is that removing particular causes of cancer from whole communities guarantees that the cancer rates will go down. If everybody stopped smoking, for example, it is a certainty that lung cancer would practically disappear in the future. Many of the other changes in behaviour and life-style which are recommended, including diet, offer less certainty in each individual case of avoiding particular cancers, but collectively they form a powerful strategy for avoiding Western diseases in general, including many of the common cancers. In the case of smoking and lung cancer a specific cause of a particular common cancer has been identified so the message is clear. Most of the other common Western cancers almost certainly have several causes which act jointly so it is important to adopt an overall strategy in your plan for avoiding them. You also have to use your common sense and have the confidence of your own convictions. No doctor can yet tell you confidently that simple actions such as taking regular exercise have been proved to help prevent particular diseases; but you are now in a position to weigh up the evidence about this and other actions for yourself. Only you can decide how much you are prepared to change your life-style to reduce your risks of getting cancer and other illnesses. Only you can decide on the balance of the evidence whether to adopt a policy which can at the least do no harm and which is most likely to do a great deal of good.

Index